THE VEGAN "BEEF" GUIDE

ALL THE ANSWERS TO WIN EVERY ARGUMENT ABOUT VEGANISM YOU WILL EVER NEED

LYANNA K. PETERSON

CONTENTS

A GIFT FOR MY READERS

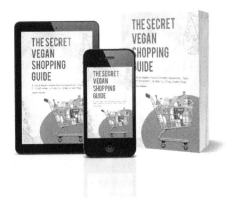

The Secret Vegan Shopping Guide

A list of hidden animal derived ingredients - from food to fashion – to help you shop cruelty fee.

Learn the truth about animal derived ingredients in your food, cosmetic products and clothing.

Could there be fish guts in your wine or animal urine in your moisturizer?

Download your free copy today and learn what ingredients you really should avoid!

Visit this link to get your copy for free:

www.the-vegan-club.com

INTRODUCTION

"Ladies, are you ready to order?"

I look up from my menu and gaze around the table.

"I'll have the pepperoni with extra cheese," says Stacey.

"And for me, the ham and pineapple please," says Belinda.

Stacey rolls her eyes. She is a big believer that pineapple does not belong on top of a pizza.

"And for you?" the waitress asks, looking over at me.

"Um, I'll just have a large mixed salad please, with balsamic dressing on the side," I fold up my menu and hand it back to the waitress.

As she leaves, I notice Stacey and Belinda staring at me.

"So, you are really going to do this vegan thing?" asks Stacey.

I nod.

"So, are you only ever going to eat salad?" asks Belinda.

"No, there are lots of things I can eat. This is just a small pizzeria with a limited menu, and they don't offer vegan cheese," I state.

"Vegan cheese?" Stacey laughs. "What is it made from nuts or something?"

"Look Lee, I know you think you are doing something good here, but in all honesty, it's not going to make a difference. It just is the circle of life. We have always eaten meat and dairy, and it's not going to change," says Belinda.

I look down at the table, not sure what I should say. Becoming vegan has become so important to me. I remember reading all these facts and figures about veganism and how it does make a huge difference but somehow, I can't put it all into simple words.

THE JOURNEY BEGINS

We live in a crazy world that has been flipped upside down. The flip appears to have affected the way people think and react. Every person has an opinion about something, and they do not realize who they hurt or offend to get their views across. It is a case of "take no prisoners" where everyone believes they have the knowledge and power to plough down whoever does not agree with them. This is something that rings true to just about every aspect of our lives, whether it be parenting, fashion, finance, or your choice of lifestyle. Instead of being supportive of people's choices, it is easier to focus on the negative aspects, make inappropriate comments, and be completely oblivious to the harm being done.

Everyone–yes, every single person who has the ability to make decisions–should be allowed to have the opportunity to have their voices heard. Sitting on the fence is something that should not be happening in this day and age. We should not have to be afraid to stand up and speak up. Arguments or differences of opinion should not end up in a full-blown battle, which is often the case. The battle of words will cause tears in the relationships between friends, family, acquaintances, or colleagues. The tongue is one of the most powerful weapons on our bodies and has the ability to inflict pain that reaches deep into our souls.

"If you can't say anything nice, don't say anything at all."

— MARGARET ATWOOD , 1976

When we are born, we do not have a voice and our parents speak and decide for us. The older we become, the more we learn how to speak up for what we want and need. We see what our peers do, and how they act. That is when we realize that we have choices. Knowing that we have choices gives us an opening to make decisions for ourselves. We become aware of our options. Whether we are ready to act on those options available to us or not, they make us think.

If we must be honest with ourselves, we have all been in a position where we have been bullied about our choices. No matter how subtle or forceful the arguments, we have all been faced with a situation where we are made to feel as if we are in the wrong.

My Story

For most of my life, meat was part of my diet. Like most meat-eating people on this earth, I never thought about a life without meat. I loved burgers and steak as much as the next person. My sister had been a vegetarian for 12 years, and no matter how many times she tried to sway me into joining her on her lifestyle journey, I stuck to my guns. I had a choice, and that choice was to continue eating meat.

In my mid-20s, I set out on a venture and travelled around Australia. To save money, I volunteered to work at a goat depot, in exchange for food and board. The guy I was working with was called Austin. He was a proper rural type of guy, strutting around in his cowboy hat and boots. Austin loved eating anything meaty and would often make fun of vegans. I do not agree with badmouthing people because yes, everyone has a right to their opinions, but to make fun of people's lifestyles does not sit well with me.

His constant joking about vegans got me thinking. Why would people choose to change their entire lifestyle? Why would they cut meat, eggs, and dairy out of their diets? Yes, my sister was a vegetarian, and I could understand her not wanting to eat a living being. We have all seen video clips and documentaries of how the animals are slaughtered. But what was wrong with consuming dairy and eggs? All these questions started stacking up, and it led me to do my own research. I watched countless documentaries on Netflix. One such documentary woke me with a jolt, and I realized that there was so much I did not know about animal agriculture.

Cowspiracy: The Sustainability Secret

The documentary that would open my eyes was, Cowspiracy: The Sustainability Secret directed by Kip Anderson and Keegan Kuhn in 2014. This documentary highlighted the effects that animal agriculture has on the environment. In addition, they explored various concerns about the environment such as global warming, deforestation, and water usage. The conclusion was made that animal farming was the main cause for the destruction of the environment.

Challenges

Following the vegan lifestyle did not come without challenges. Although I was one of the lucky ones, and have a supportive family, my dad who is a big meat eater, would often challenge me at mealtimes. The comments ranged from "there is not enough farmland to grow fruit and vegetables to feed the entire population" to "eating soy is destroying the rainforest". Being new to the lifestyle, I did not have all the answers to counteract his comments. Even though I love a good discussion with my dad, constantly not having a good answer left me feeling deflated. Not only did I lose the argument, but I also lost a valuable chance of making him change his mind or reconsider veganism being something serious and not just a fad.

No matter what we do in life, we will always be faced with challenges. There will always be those that do not understand why we are following a lifestyle that does not fit in with the ideas of others. We can always try to get our views across, but unless the other person has an open mind, we will be walking into brick walls. The best we can do is to equip people with the necessary knowledge without being forceful and allow them to decide for themselves.

EDUCATION IS KEY

It is so easy to judge a book by its cover without reading the words between the covers. This is what life is like. Everyone has an opinion without understanding or wanting to understand the reasons. Everyone jumps to a conclusion that has no relevance to the situation.

People will throw all types of arguments in your direction, and I want you to be able to have the confidence to counteract those arguments with grace and confidence. You will encounter people who will be downright nasty about your lifestyle, but you will be able to stand up for yourself and argue your case.

A New Vision

It is no secret that we are living in trying times. The world as we knew it has changed and we have had to adapt to our new way of life. We should re-evaluate our lifestyles to fit in with the new norm. If the global pandemic taught us anything, it was that the environment had time to recover when everyone was forced to stay home. The beaches have never been cleaner, the skies brighter, and the air purer than during the lockdown.

In this guide, you will find examples I came across when I started on my new lifestyle journey. I am passionate about veganism and I want to help others see that they will be benefiting. Whether this is a new venture or a refresher crash course, we are going to have our voices heard and we will be giving stragglers the motivation that they need.

Put on your most comfortable sweats, don a pair of fluffy socks, shoes optional, and let us start exploring and appreciating what our wonderful earth has to offer. Together, one person at a time, we can make a difference.

1

UNDERSTANDING VEGANISM

The human mind is like a sponge. It has and continues to absorb every bit of information we have been given. From the time we are born, we are learning. As we grow up, we remember what we have been taught by our parents, grandparents, teachers, and everyone around us. We even remember the little things we should not have heard and save them for the day where we can string sentences together. No one thought to ask us what we wanted during our formative years.

The same can be said for changing your lifestyle. When your mind is made up, and you decide what you want, you do the research, read the articles, surf the internet, or ask questions. Once you have decided what is best for you, you inform those nearest and dearest to you of your intentions. They are either supportive or look at you as if you have lost your mind.

How can you expect someone to understand and be supportive of your choices when they do not know the history? Whether it is a seed that is planted or a great past event that sets the course of our future, everything has to start somewhere. The vegan lifestyle, amongst others, is no different. Veganism is not some kind of lifestyle that was conjured up because someone woke up one day and decided to stop eating meat and animal by-products.

THE HISTORY OF VEGANISM

"A journey of a thousand miles begins with a single step."

— CHINESE PROVERB

If we want to fully understand the vegan lifestyle, we are going to have to take a stroll through the archives. History might not be everyone's favourite, but it is a subject that holds the answers to many questions. Love it or hate it, history is a part of our genetic make-up. Whether we care to admit it or not, history plays a massive role in how our future is shaped. People and events make it into the history books and are subjects taught at school. Without discrediting the past, nowhere was something as important as diet, lifestyle, parenting, or fashion choices featured in our school books. Unless you were looking for something specific, you would have to dig very deep to follow the breadcrumbs to get you the answers that you would need.

The Beginning

Without having a name or definition until the late 1900s, the exclusion of animal and animal by-products, and an exclusively vegetarian lifestyle dates back to 500 BCE. Although the lifestyle did not have a name, it was believed to have been a vegetarian diet. Pythagoras, the Greek philosopher, and mathematician encouraged the lifestyle that represented kindness and compassion amongst people and animals. The vegetarian lifestyle was also part of spiritual and religious practices, such as Buddhism.

In approximately 1806, Dr. William Lambe and Percy Bysshe Shelley stood up for what they believed in, which was opposing the consumption of eggs and dairy. Their reasoning for their choice was based on the grounds of ethical morals. It was believed that the duo prepared the world for what would, in the future, become the vegan lifestyle.

Donald Watson

November 1944 saw a group consisting of six like-minded people sit down together to discuss the plight of the vegetarian diet and lifestyle. The group was trying to define their vegetarian diet which excluded consuming animal by-products. The group, led by Mr. Donald Watson, was adamant in giving their plant-based diet a new name by removing it from the vegetarian branding.

They were met with opposition by non-members, but the group pushed through and stood their ground. Between them, they decided on a new name for the 'new' lifestyle. A number of names were thrown around until Donald came up with a solution that would become a name everyone would get to know– the first three and last two letters of the word 'vegetarian' which spelled 'vegan'. Not only was the term vegan coined, but it was also the birth of The Vegan Society which is still in operation in 2021.

Leslie J. Cross

Thanks to Mr. Donald Watson, the original group concluded that there had to be a split between the two lifestyles, followers of the lifestyle would be able to define their diets. Unfortunately, Leslie J. Cross was not content with the idea of separating the vegetarian and vegan lifestyles. He wanted The Vegan Society to have a plausible definition, something other than "eating a plant-based diet and preserving animals and animal by-products" type of definition.

Leslie Cross was appointed as the vice-president of The Vegan Society in 1949, and it was during this that he came up with a definition for the word 'veganism', as well as an objective for what the society stands for.

"The word veganism shall mean the doctrine that man should live without exploiting animals" and "The object of the Society shall be to end the exploitation of animals by man".

— LESLIE CROSS , 1951.

The Vegan Society

For the last leg, our history lesson will be looking at The Vegan Society which was founded in the United Kingdom in 1944. The Vegan Society was the first official society in the world that was dedicated to the vegan lifestyle. It has grown and evolved since the Donald Watson and Leslie Cross days.

The original society was registered as a charity in 1964. After 15 years, in 1979, The Vegan Society became a limited company and charity organization. The definition and objectives of The Vegan Society changed over the space of 20-odd years to keep up with the changing times. An updated version of the objectives and definition was released in 1988, which would be used in the current day and age.

"In this memorandum, the word 'veganism' denotes a philosophy and way of living which seeks to exclude–as far as is possible and practicable–all forms of exploitation of, and cruelty, to animals for food, clothing or any other purpose; and by extension, promotes the development and use of animal-free alternatives for the benefit of humans, animals, and the environment. In dietary terms, it denoted the practice of dispensing with all products derived wholly or partly from animals." – The Vegan Society, 1988.

WHY CHOOSE A VEGAN LIFESTYLE?

"It is not enough to be compassionate. You must act."

— DALAI LAMA

The moment you mention that you are considering adopting the vegan lifestyle, or if you are already following it, people jump on their little pedestals. Instead of asking questions, they add their own interpretation and hit you with misguided facts that they probably heard from someone who heard it along the grapevine. It does not matter who says what, but at the end of the day, the one that is going to be affected is the one trying to justify why they are doing what they are doing. This is not something that is exclusive to following a vegan lifestyle, this occurs in all aspects of our lives.

Every year, polls are conducted to establish where the population stands in terms of following trends, which diets they follow, and what their preferred choice of lifestyle is. In January 2021, it was determined that the approximate vegan population throughout the world stands proudly at 79 million people. In a world with over 7 billion inhabitants, 79 million might seem like an insignificant number. If you compare the statistics from 2019 to January of 2021, it is safe to say that over a two-year period, the vegan population more than tripled.

The growth period over the two years has proven that veganism is on the increase. People are becoming more aware of what they are doing to the earth. Maybe a little prod from the world in crisis helped people see a little clearer and inspired the change, no one will really know. One thing that we can hold onto, is that if the vegan community continues to grow at the current rate, veganism might just become the preferred lifestyle in the next 30 years.

There are many reasons why people choose to follow the vegan lifestyle. We will look at some of the main reasons.

Compassion for the Animals

Most people are aware of what happens in slaughterhouses. They are fully aware of the gruesome acts that take place. They will never admit this to anyone, especially to vegans, so they pretend to overlook these atrocities. Not many people are aware of what happens on dairy farms or egg farms. The question of whether being a vegetarian, which we will debunk later in the book, is not enough.

We have all been to the circus as children, been entertained by dolphins performing tricks, or seen shows where animals are put on display for our entertainment. Winter sees us donning thick woolly jumpers, knitted mittens, and leather boots lined with fur. We also use the down feathers from ducks in our duvets. Women apply foundation, lipstick, eye shadow, eyeliner, and mascara with the utmost precision to make them look good for a night out with the girls or that special someone in our lives.

Those leather boots cost a cow its life. The wool we wear is obtained when the sheep are sheared in spring. We tend to believe what we see in the television shows where the handsome shearers pick up a sheep, holds it down, and starts shearing and pats its rear as he is released. In reality, the sheep are traumatized and hurt during the shearing season. The feathers for our duvets are plucked from the ducks while they are alive, thereby torturing them.

The make-up we so lovingly applied was manufactured by doing cruel tests on animals in laboratories. Thanks to the global pandemic, every single human on this earth knows what it is like to be 'locked' up at home for months on end. No one ever thought the tables would be turned when we became animals in our homes. Imagine exchanging places with the animals living in the zoos or circuses, where they are caged or fenced in.

By changing our lifestyles, and adopting the vegan lifestyle, we are going to try to stop all forms of abuse to animals.

Health

When people find out that you are a vegan, they start telling you that you are depriving your body of the necessary nutrients only animal products and by-products can give you. If I had a dollar for every time someone said that to me, I would have bought an island and populated it with all the animals I could fit.

Every diet or lifestyle poses a health risk. If you eat meat and dairy, you stand the risk of getting cancer, high blood pressure, or high cholesterol. This is a topic that will get everyone talking. Vegans, although not immune to any health issues, are less likely to attract such illnesses because they have made the conscious decision to eliminate animal products from their diets. They are less likely to suffer from debilitating diseases such as diabetes, heart disease, osteoporosis, or obesity (Sinrich, 2021).

Animal Agriculture and Climate Change

Everyone agrees that the climate is not what it was 20-odd years ago. Countries are experiencing a range of bizarre weather conditions which are brushed off as "acts of nature." Droughts, earthquakes, extreme snowstorms, and flash flooding have been reported all across the globe. Yes, these are acts of nature, but it is nature fighting to survive. Every single person on this planet has had a hand in breaking down the environment. First and foremost is the farming of animals for food.

Animal agriculture is the leading cause of climate change causing 51% of greenhouse gas emissions. This accounts for at least 32 million tons of carbon dioxide each year (Hickman, 2009).

Ruminant animals such as cows, sheep, and goats also produce a gas known as methane. This gas is approximately 25 times more powerful than carbon dioxide. According to an article written for the BBC by Geoff Watts in August of 2019, cows and sheep produce an average of 250 litres to 500 litres of methane per day. The methane being released from livestock across the world equates to a staggering 3.1 gigatons per year (Watts, 2019).

All of these gases stop the heat of the world from leaving the atmosphere. You can imagine this like a big bubble around the world trapping the heat inside the bubble. This is known as the "greenhouse" effect.

Right now, most of the extra heat is getting absorbed by our oceans. This is causing the temperature of the water to rise which in turn is responsible for the ice melting. The melting of the ice has a huge impact on our wildlife and coastal life. When the ice melts, it causes sea levels to rise and if this continues, it means that cities and towns in and around the coastlines will be underwater.

Any changes to the sea can cause extreme droughts, floods, and even wildfires. This means that the land that is used to produce crops for food will suffer because of the lack of water, flooding, and destruction. Communities cannot live and thrive in certain areas anymore as the land becomes too hostile. The International Organization for Migration (IOM), has predicted that the world will have between 150 and 200 million climate refugees by 2050 (Kamal, 2017).

If we look at some figures based on a study done in 2018, non-vegans should be thinking twice before biting into that piece of rump steak or indulging in that three-egg omelette. Looking at the global position of agricultural land, 83% is used for animal agriculture.

The land is used to grow crops and raise animals for human consumption. What many people do not want to see is that raising these animals takes a lot more than fattening them up.

There is a ripple effect and when the ripple comes to an end, it begins again.

The land needs to be cleared to plant crops for the animals. The land needs fertilizer to ensure that the crops provide sufficient food. The crops need water to grow. More often than not, the crops are sprayed with insecticide which the animals ingest. When the animals are fattened up, they are sent to the abattoirs. Logging machinery and the transport vehicles used to transport the animals emit carbon monoxide. At the slaughterhouses, the animals are slaughtered. Fecal matter and blood are washed away with water. The runoff ends up in the water table below the ground. The tainted water seeps into the bodies of water. Water animals are affected by the water. People are affected.

Deforestation

We know that when we breathe, we are filling our lungs with oxygen which is vitally important to humans and animals to survive. Our bodies need oxygen, as well as food, to keep us energized. When we exhale the depleted oxygen, we are clearing our lungs of carbon dioxide. The carbon dioxide that we exhale is now absorbed by the plants and trees around us. The beauty of nature steps in and the trees and plants use carbon dioxide to make their own energy, which means they do not need to eat.

Trees and plants have a purpose for the environment. In a world where the population consists of over 7 billion people, trees are needed to absorb all the carbon dioxide, as well as all the other gases that are emitted to purify the air we breathe in. Along comes man and his need to profit off the manufacturing of animal products. To achieve his ultimate goal and need for greed, the forests and vegetation that are needed to keep a healthy balance for the environment and ecosystem are broken down. The trees are cut down to make room for more land for animal farming.

Pollution

As I have mentioned, life as we knew it came to a standstill due to the global pandemic in 2020. The whole world's population was given orders to stay home. Some countries enforced these orders with the help of the military, and others trusted their inhabitants to adhere to the new laws. In most countries, surfing, swimming, and walks along the beach were not permitted. Driving to work or traveling for pleasure or business was prohibited. People were forced to work from home, thereby reducing the number of harmful gases in the atmosphere. For the better part of nine months, the environment and ecosystem were given a new lease on life, as it was allowed to recover from decades' worth of pollution.

Pollution does not only occur because of littering or the emission of harmful gases into the atmosphere. Slaughterhouses, factories, production plants, and all enterprises involved in the manufacturing of packaging and food handling all contribute to the breakdown of the environment. Animal agriculture not only has a negative impact on dry land, it adversely impacts the oceans too.

Every animal and critter has been created for a purpose, but instead of living the life that was intended for them, they are running scared because their safe havens are being destroyed. Our oceans and sea life, which include fish, sharks, whales, dolphins, and turtles are finding themselves under stress, and many are facing extinction or are already extinct due to pollution and overfishing.

As hard as it is to imagine, even the ocean and sea life need oxygen to survive. Sadly, due to the ongoing mass production of animal agriculture and the processes involved, the ocean is being suffocated. The amount of pollution that makes its way into the water table on the surface of the earth, and then leaks into the bodies of water such as rivers, lakes, and oceans, is causing areas to be declared as dead zones. These dead zones are detrimental to our environment as they are responsible for the lack of oxygen in our oceans.

Overfishing is another serious threat to our environment. Over half of the plastic found in our oceans is from plastic fishing nets. A large number of species are facing extinction as they are caught and killed by commercial fishers and trawlers. It is important to note that our oceans are vital in the prevention of climate change. It is believed that more than 70% of the carbon dioxide emissions will end up in the ocean (Shutler & Watson, 2020). A healthy fish population is extremely important to our oceans.

In an article by Candy Belle in October of 2020 for an online website, scientists have predicted that our oceans could be fishless by 2048. The study was conducted by an international team of economists and ecologists (Belle, 2020). What many people do not realize or understand, is that the oceans are vital to our existence. If the ocean dies, we will die (Watson, 2015).

ARE YOU READY?

I can go on for days and present you with hundreds of reasons why you should follow the vegan lifestyle, but it is not you that I need to convince. You know what you want, but all that you need now is the courage to have your voice heard. Stand firm in what you believe in, be confident in yourself and allow your passion for the world to tumble out of your mouth with grace. You do not have to earn brownie points from friends or family for what you believe in. Your passion comes from a place where you have compassion and empathy for any and all living and breathing creatures.

2

BRIDGING THE DEFENSIVE BARRIER

The subject of veganism is often treated like politics and religion. Not everyone will agree with your views. Even though I don't believe it is ok to reduce the concept of animal abuse to a difference of opinion, unless people are open-minded and willing to listen to reasoning, you cannot force them to change their habits. People are afraid of making changes. Decades of believing that their way is the right way will require patience to help them understand what a change could do for them. We are going to explore some of the most common reasons why people become defensive when being presented with the idea of becoming vegan.

One has to laugh at people's reactions when they are told that you are vegan. It is as though everyone suddenly becomes a doctor or nutritionist thanks to the medical school of Google.

Most arguments that are presented are misguided. Reading a blog that someone wrote based on a hearsay conversation about a vegan who became malnourished because they were not getting the required proteins and nutrients that can only be found in meat has us rolling our eyes. If only they knew that there were better and healthier options than consuming animal products.

In chapter 4, we will delve into more of the arguments that we, as vegans, are faced with. No matter what diet or dietary lifestyle you decide to follow, you will always have the Google medical graduates telling you about all the negative side effects and ignoring the benefits.

Why are many meat eaters defensive when in the company of vegans? Why do they feel so threatened by the idea of not eating meat? Let us explore some ideas to see why they are so afraid to entertain the vegan lifestyle.

Identity

What is a man without his manly steak? It is believed that our forefathers, dating back to the cavemen age, hunted for their food. Through the centuries, the mentality of the hunter was passed on from generation to generation. In many social scenarios, men are known to man the barbecue that puts perfectly cooked steaks, pork chops, or chicken on the plates. Barbecues are also the social gathering place for the men who are enjoying a drink and cooking for their guests. In this instance, one can almost understand why they will feel conflicted with the vegan lifestyle.

Men, especially, are afraid of changing their meat-eating habits for that of a plant-based diet. People are generally afraid of any type of change. Some are afraid that changes would bring about endless teasing if they were to cook cauliflower steaks on the barbecue instead of a thick slab of meat. Choosing a plant-based diet over a meat-based diet might take away their identity of being manly men.

I get why people are afraid to change. What people seem to forget is that times have changed. The population has sky-rock-eted to a point where more land is used to build houses to accommodate the ever-growing population, more land is used to grow crops to feed more animals, and more animals are produced to feed everyone. No one was able to foresee what the global population would be like 50-plus years into the future. We need to stop thinking about what people think about us and think about what is best for our environment.

Criticism

Referring back to the Introduction, when I went out for lunch with Belinda and Stacey. I opted for the salad because the restaurant did not have a vegan menu. When I did not choose a pizza off the menu, I might have subconsciously been sending out vibes that eating meat and dairy is not acceptable and by doing so, they may have felt as if I was criticizing their lifestyle choices.

As much as people like living in their own bubbles, I do believe that deep down, everyone knows that the way animals are treated is wrong. Everyone watches documentaries, reads articles, and hears stories. By seeing other people acting upon things that they know they should also be doing, but do not want to do, it can make them feel resentful towards you. Being the first person in my friend circle to make a change, I do believe I am giving my friends the courage to see that I am not bothered by what society thinks of me and I hope to give them the courage to do the same.

Whether they walked away from our lunch date wondering if I was trying to convert them or condemn them for their choices, is a question only they can answer. I have never forced my beliefs on anyone, and I am not going to start now. I am trying to show friends and family, with respect, that what I believe in means a lot to me.

Tactlessness

The shields come up when people feel that they are being attacked for their choices. We encounter people from all walks of life. No two people in the world are the same, and everyone has the free will to decide what is best for them. When crossing paths with someone who does not share your choices, it is only right to be respectful. Vegans are passionate about the journey they are on. Meat-eaters are passionate about their dietary choices.

As vegans, we can be very emotional about our beliefs and we can be quick to say tactless things. Telling a meat-eater that he is a murderer can never be the start of a productive conversation as they could become defensive. We must remember that meat-eaters are not bad people. They are just doing what they have been taught to do since they were little. It is important to remember that at some point in our lives we also ate meat, dairy, and eggs because we did not know any better.

Feeling Overwhelmed

When faced with the option of changing your dietary lifestyle, you are met with trepidation. Some people make the choice to change in the blink of an eye, and others sit there with their lists of pros and cons. It is a scary thought, for meat-eaters, to change their eating habits. When they are faced with questions from their friends or family about what their diet would look like, they are fearful, thinking that they will never eat 'proper' food again.

Most people who hear about the vegan lifestyle think that dinner will be a plate of cooked vegetables, a salad on the side, and a slice of dry bread for example. Not many realize that veganism has evolved over the years, and the options for plant-based diets are plentiful. All plant-based foods are responsibly sourced and contain a healthy balance of nutrients and vitamins.

As vegans, it is up to us to help the lonely meat-eater and guide them through the process. We need to be patient with them. We do not want to overwhelm them with our knowledge until they are ready to make the change themselves. Be ready with the answers to their questions- and they will have questions. They will be relaying the information to their loved ones to help them understand that they will not be starving.

We now have a little more of an understanding of why meat-eaters put up defensive barriers when confronted by vegans. It is up to us to help them, guide them, and allow them to set the course. We need to be subtle in our approach. We need to show compassion for them. Even if they are still following their chosen dietary lifestyle, we can show them that there are options.

We want the world to see that vegans are not bullies. While there might be a handful of extremists who do go a little too far, not everyone is the same. There are some tender-hearted vegans. Some would even go as far as to say that meat-eaters "hate us". Hate is such a small word that is filled with so much anger and resentment. I would like to believe that meat-eaters do not hate vegans, but they are afraid of being judged for their choices. In a world that is filled with so much controversy that affects every aspect of our lives, it is time for all of us to stand together. We have the ability to make the world we live in a better place, even if it is just one small change a week.

3

COMMUNICATION WITHOUT CONFRONTATION

C ommunication is an important part of our existence. Many will say that they talk to their pets or plants and that they do not need people. It is all good and well to talk to our pets or plants because they do not talk back or judge us. We are well aware that people like to pick an argument without listening to reason. The truth of the matter is, we need people. Sometimes, communicating with people can be daunting and overwhelming, especially when you are an introvert or if you do not care to get into an argument.

Communication is healthy for our existence. Everyone needs someone to talk to, bounce ideas off, or a sympathetic ear who will listen to us. Many people will withdraw from a confrontation and bite their tongues rather than argue with someone they care about. Others will dive in and say what is on their mind, often saying something that has no relevance to the original conversation. We cannot please everyone, but we can also not be quiet when something is important to us. Is it possible to discuss something important and meaningful to us without ending up in a word-slinging battle? Yes, it is. We have the power to have our voices heard without being mean.

COMMUNICATION PITFALLS

When we feel that we are not being heard, we take it personally. We feel like school children who are being dismissed for having an opinion. We walk away from the situation with anger and frustration because we also want a little piece of the sun that everyone is supposed to share. We allow these feelings to fester until one day, someone will say something that does not sit well with you, and you let it all out.

Emotions

Emotions play a big role in how we communicate with people. When you are feeling stressed, angry, or overwhelmed, your emotions are heightened. Many times, it just takes someone to look at you or say something to you for you to become verbal. I get it. There is only so much prodding and teasing you can take before you say something you will regret.

When you find yourself in a position where your emotions are threatening to overwhelm you, take a step back. Breathe in deeply and exhale. Count to 10. If you feel like you cannot face the situation, take a walk. Always remember that when you say something hurtful to someone, you can never take those words back.

"Sticks and stones may break our bones, but words will break our hearts."

— ROBERT FULGHUM

Distractions

If you are having a conversation with someone, they may pick up when they do not have your full attention. To effectively communicate with someone, you need to focus on that person. If they notice that you are not listening to what they are saying, they could potentially blindside you with their opinion before you can turn that situation around.

When you are talking to someone, focus on what they are saying. People are proud to say that they have a degree in multi-tasking, but when you are in company, you need to put that skill to bed. Always be prepared for the unexpected and stay focused.

Body Language

Your body language tells a person how you really feel about a situation. If you are having a conversation with someone you do not like, they can read the signs. The way you act tells the other person how you really feel. Even if you are agreeing with what is being said, your body language will tell the person your true feelings. It is safe to say that some people are oblivious and only hear what they want to hear. No matter what the situation or the conversation is about, you want to be honest in your communication.

The same could be said for being negative. If you do not agree with someone's opinion, your energy will alert them to your true feelings. By avoiding eye contact, fidgeting, moving around, crossing your arms, or feeling uncomfortable, you will send out signals of negativity. No matter how uncomfortable you are feeling with the conversation, practice your breathing and remain calm. Think happy thoughts and listen to the other person without judgment. When the opportunity presents itself for you to have your say, do so without negative thoughts.

HOW TO APPROACH MEAT-EATERS AND HAVE YOUR VOICE HEARD

I know you are eagerly waiting to go out and share your passion for the vegan lifestyle with everyone. You need to practice restraint and patience, especially when it comes to bridging the communication barriers. What you want is to approach people without overwhelming them. You do not want to ambush them, become defensive and then open the door to an argument without having stated your case.

You want to speak to meat-eaters, and you want them to listen to you and your reasons for becoming a vegan. By the time you reach the end of this chapter, you will know how to draw in a tough cookie and have them eating a veggie burger–we are allowed to hope.

Find Common Ground

Most people are pet owners, having any number of dogs, cats, or any other animal. While not all people treat their pets as a part of their family, they nevertheless are most likely to oppose animal cruelty. When starting a conversation with someone, refer to their love for animals. This will make your opponent feel more comfortable and understood. This will lead to a much more positive and constructive conversation.

Simplicity

I know we are passionate about our vegan lifestyle, but we are not selling a product. Do not present people with all the nitty-gritty facts and statistics. You want to connect with people on a personal level. Keep it simple. Tell them why the vegan lifestyle is so important to you. Be ready with answers to questions that may follow.

Do Not Expect A Change Straight Away

Some people take a little longer to make a decision than others, so do not set the bar of expectation too high. If they tell you that they will do their own research, accept their response. Do not needle them into giving you an answer and expect transformation right away. Allow the person to walk away, knowing that you gave a stellar testimony. Be positive that they will change.

Be Honest

When speaking to someone, make sure that you have the relevant information you want to convey. Let the people you are talking to know why you are passionate about being a vegan. Be honest, because people can tell when you are lying, and if you are trying to win someone over, you will lose that person before you have stated your case. Present them with the information you have gathered. Speak about what is personal to you, not your friends or your family, but yourself.

No Judgment

No one knows what the other person is going through, or what they have gone through to get to the position they are presently at. The same can be said for meat-eaters. We need to understand that if we are going to attack them for their choices, we will have lost someone who could have been instrumental in being the voice of veganism.

If you want to win someone over, you have to do so without nit-picking, judgment, undue pressure, and guilt trips. You have done what you could to get your point across, now leave it and stop trying to get a response from them. They will approach you with questions in their own time.

No Shame

As much as you would like to believe that you are a walking encyclopedia, or a mobile version of Google, remember that you are just a regular human being. As long as you are speaking from your heart and relating your personal experience, all will be okay. Remember that you do not always have to have a smart comeback right away. You can tell your opponent that you will have to think about it and then bring the conversation back to the topics you are confident with.

Throwing In the Towel

Do not get yourself into a situation where you are going to feel trapped for sharing your story. Even if you cannot sway one person, just remember that you have planted a seed. Over time, the seed will grow and it will take shape somewhere during the person's life. Do not stand around and allow anyone to badmouth you because of your choice. You have to assess when to walk away from a situation.

WINNING ONE ARGUMENT AT A TIME

"Strong people stand up for themselves, but stronger people stand up for others."

— SUZY KASSEM

The Socrates Method

Dating back to between 470 and 399 BC, an ancient Greek philosopher by the name of Socrates hailed from Athens. It is believed that Socrates never documented his work in text, therefore there is no official written work from him. His preferred method of sharing his work was by teaching his students and passing on his moral philosophy. Socrates has many students such as Plato, Xenophon, and Aristophanes. It was thanks to Plato, that Socrates' work was able to be heard and incorporated into the teaching of many over the centuries.

Socrates developed a method of having a conversation or argument with someone using a specialized dialogue. The technique allows for a question to be asked and gives the opponent the chance to think about his answer. The thinking period will also allow for the opponent to reach a conclusion without having someone tell them what the answer should be. The principle of the Socratic Method is to allow your opponent to form their own ideas, as well as see both sides of the coin without being forced to choose between white and black, or if the glass is half full or half empty.

If you want to win arguments, you are going to have to let the people believe they have come to the conclusion themselves. You are going to allow people to think for themselves by asking them questions. There are no right or wrong answers. We are not going to spoon-feed people into thinking one way, but instead, give them the choice to form their own opinions and make their own decisions based on the types of questions they are faced with.

Everyone is going to think their method of asking questions is the right way. Some will take a long time to get to the question as they are testing the waters and possibly assessing the person's attitude or temper. Others will go in straight for the jugular, and there is no stopping the temper from exploding. I believe that people are tired of skirting around a subject. It is time to be open, honest, and straightforward, but not forceful to the point of chasing someone away.

There are two main types of questions that you can use on your opponent: open and closed lines of questions.

Closed questions can only be answered with yes or no. Your opponent does not have to think much and it keeps you in control of where the conversation is going.

We can also ask open lines of questions that cannot be answered with a simple yes or no. These questions make your opponent think and share their opinion.

In my experience, it is best to start a conversation with a closed question. As the conversation starts flowing, you can move on to more open questions.

Example:

I would start by asking my opponent: "Do you believe animal cruelty is wrong?"
Usually, the person would answer with: "Yes."
I would then move on and ask them: "Why do you believe animal cruelty is wrong?"
At this point, it is important to validate what the person is saying.
I would then continue the conversation by asking: "Would you deem stealing a baby away from its mother as cruel, and if you do, why?"
Next, I would say: "In the dairy industry, baby calves are taken away from their mothers only hours after giving birth. Would you agree that this is animal cruelty?"

Open and closed questions both have value. I feel that it is best to use both to keep the conversation flowing easily.

4

EXCUSE ME THIS, EXCUSE ME THAT, EXCUSES DEBUNKED ALL OVER THE PLACE

"First they ignore you, then they laugh at you, then they fight you, then you win."

— UNKNOWN

Everyone makes excuses. It is a part of our coping mechanism for wanting to avoid difficult or uncomfortable situations. Some people believe that coming up with excuses is the perfect solution to protect themselves against being embarrassed. It is sad that society has made the use of excuses necessary. Instead of saying no and giving a valid reason, we often validate our 'no' with an excuse.

As you know, this guide is all about equipping you with the knowledge that is needed to debunk people's common misconceptions about following the vegan lifestyle. Until now, you have racked up all the important facts that you can use to tell people about the vegan lifestyle. You know how to enter into a conversation and diffuse an argument by asking some open-ended questions that will make your opponent think.

Human beings, like animals, are curious by nature. Once a seed has been planted, they will be thinking and wondering about what comes next. You need to be ready for any and all questions they will come back with. That is why I have prepared a list of the possible questions and excuses they will have, as well as answers to help them understand. As far as excuses go, there are always ways to counter them with valid responses. Now without further ado, let's get started.

SOY FARMING IS RUINING THE RAINFOREST

One of the first arguments I often hear is that vegans are responsible for the destruction of the rainforests. They will continue their argument by telling us that we are so passionate about saving the environment and the animals, that we overlook the fact that it is our food that is responsible.

If it were true that all the soy crops that are being planted and harvested for the production of plant-based foods, then I would accept responsibility. Yes, the environment is impacted by soy farming, but it is important to remember that vegans are not the only ones that eat soy. In fact, if you were to do research, you would discover that between 70% and 85% of the global production of soy is distributed among the factory farms. Keep an eye on the person's face you are talking to when you inform them that only 6% of the soy is used for food for human consumption. The remainder of the soy is made into soybean oil (Good, 2015).

You could ask the person using this excuse: "If you are concerned about soy farming, along with the environmental impact, would you give up consuming animal products knowing that 70% to 85% is used as food for the animals you are eating?"

I love it when meat eaters say that they will never eat soy products. These are obviously people who do not read the ingredients on the packages with a magnifying glass! When it is said that 6% of the soy that is harvested becomes food, it does not mean that it will be made into vegan products. Non-vegan products contain soy, and unless people are diagnosed with a soy allergy, they may be oblivious to the fact that they are enjoying their favourite foods with trace amounts of soy. You will find soy in many soups, cereals, cookies, chocolate, crackers, processed meats, and baked goods.

As a side note, vegans do not necessarily eat soy products. It might sound as though we are restricted by the food we consume, but there are many more plant-based foods to enjoy.

Let the people you are talking to understand why their ideology about the soy farming industry and veganism is warped. Remind them that one to two acres of forestation is cleared every second to create more land for the animal agriculture industry. As we have previously seen when addressing the climate change issue, animal agriculture accounts for up to 51% of greenhouse gas emissions.

When addressing the climate crisis in August 2019, a panel of researchers commissioned by the United Nations Organization notes that the answer to the problem is on our plates. It is suggested that people should change their diets to that of a plant-based one.

End the conversation by stating: "If you claim to truly care about the environment and the effects of climate change, then you should do something proactive and become a vegan."

HUMAN BEINGS ARE MORE INTELLIGENT THAN ANIMALS

As human beings, we pride ourselves on being the most intelligent species alive. We tend to place ourselves on a pedestal that allows us to believe that we are more superior. This thought process justifies us taking the lives of billions of animals.

The truth of the matter is that we cannot compare our intelligence to animals because they are more intelligent than we give them credit for.

Have you ever heard of an animal destroying its habitat?

We are destroying the only home we know at an alarming rate. We are responsible for cutting down the rainforests, polluting the oceans, and our skies. Some might argue that they do not participate in these acts. Whether directly or indirectly, we are contributing. How can we call ourselves intelligent human beings?

If the person you are talking to says it is okay to eat pigs because they are less intelligent than humans, for the sake of the argument, should we not be eating animals that are the least intelligent species or less intelligent than pigs?

Did you know that pigs are highly intelligent animals? When we think of pigs, we picture them living in muddy fenced-in designated areas of farms. Pigs make excellent pets, as they are easily trained because they have excellent memories. They learn their names and tricks faster than a puppy. They are very proud animals that do not sleep near their food troughs or bathroom area. They do not sweat and therefore roll around in the mud to keep cool. People often mistakenly believe that pigs are dirty and smelly. Pigs are believed to be on the same cognitive level as a three-year-old child.

Thinking about this example again, if we should eat less intelligent animals, should we not be eating dogs instead?

What this argument boils down to is, what does intelligence have to do with the life of an animal? Why would someone less intelligent deserve less in life? Present your opponent with these questions. Then ask them: "Do you believe that just because someone is smarter than you, they should have the right to dominate over your life?" If the response is no, then ask them: "Why is it okay for us to treat animals in that way?"

GOD CREATED ANIMALS TO BE EATEN

The bible consists of 66 books, 39 in the Old Testament and 27 in the New Testament. In total, there are 31,102 verses in the bible. It is no secret that people quote from the bible to suit themselves, and only seem to read what they want to be heard. There are those who will dispute the creation to turn it around to please them. This book is not based on an argument of who said what and who did what. We are here for the voiceless because we want to protect all living creatures.

For the sake of the argument, let us agree that God created animals. Nowhere in the bible does it say that we HAVE to eat meat. There is also no religion that tells us that we have to eat meat, nor refrain from eating meat. Day three saw the creation of plants and trees. Days five and six saw the creation of sea life, winged animals, and land animals, as well as man. Nowhere does it say that man has to hunt animals for pleasure or profit.

Even If it was necessary to consume meat, eggs, and dairy in biblical times, the world has evolved, and the population has multiplied by over a million. We live in a world of convenience where we have multiple options available to us. You can walk into a store and buy whatever you want or with a click of a button have your groceries delivered to your door.

Something you could ask your opponent is: "In a world where it is so easily accessible to eat meat and dairy alternatives, why would you choose to unnecessarily kill a creature created by God?"

God created all animals for a certain purpose and in a certain way. Humans have genetically modified animals to produce more milk and eggs, to grow faster and bigger, with the main reason to increase profits and demand. Humans have intervened in the natural process of life and by doing so are playing God themselves. There were no scientists in biblical times, and the animals God created were free to roam and be animals.

Something else you could ask the person you are talking to is: "Do you believe that God would be happy with the way we have genetically modified his animals?"

If you have watched documentaries or YouTube videos showing how animals are artificially inseminated, genetically modified, physically and mentally abused, before being carted off to the slaughterhouses you will have seen the fear and pain on those animals' faces.

To end the conversation, leave the person with the following question: "Do you believe that this is what a kind and compassionate God intended when he created animals?"

ANIMALS EAT OTHER ANIMALS

This statement always makes me laugh. Many people believe, because we are animals, we can behave like animals.

The truth is you cannot compare human behaviour to animal behaviour. Humans act because they put thought into the action. Animals act on their instinct to survive, and that is why they eat other animals. In the animal kingdom, many animals will kill other animals and sometimes they will kill their offspring.

Based on the knowledge we have about the animal kingdom, such as killing their young, you could ask the person you are talking to: "Do you believe it is wise to base our actions on animal behaviour?"

If you have ever watched nature shows like Animal Planet, you would have seen how wild animals interact with each other in their natural habitat. You have seen the lion or the hyena chase after their prey. By using their instinct, they immobilize their prey by biting into their throats. This is what happens in nature, between animals, to survive.

I want you to visualize a scenario where you are looking through a window and you see a pig roaming around. Not too far from the pig, you see a lion prowling. The lion is watching the pig with interest. The lion suddenly realizes that he is hungry and instinct tells him that this is a meal ticket for his pride. He pounces on the pig. Using his teeth and claws, he kills the pig and tears into the flesh. Lions are not picky eaters, and they will eat everything, from the snout to the tail, and everything in between. Lions love the smell of raw flesh and blood because that is their instinct.

If I had to switch places with the lion, and I saw the pig, I would approach it carefully so as not to startle it. I would be armed with nothing but my two hands and not so sharp set of teeth to go in for the kill. He will look at me as if I am slightly crazy, and then assume that I want to play with him because there is no possible way I would be able to, using the only 'weapons' I have, kill him. All I would end up doing is tickling his belly and having a giggle as he grunts in pleasure. Without weapons, we would have no chance to kill the pig. I believe we can safely say that we are not lions, so we should not act like lions.

The human body is not made to eat raw animal flesh. Eating raw meat, such as pork, can make us feel sick, as well as cause a whole host of medical issues such as food poisoning and tapeworms

(Marengo, 2020). Our bodies differ greatly from those of animals. Our digestive system does not produce enough acid to break down the animal flesh.

Something you could ask your opponent is: "How do you feel when you see violent images of animals being killed, such as in slaughterhouse footage?"

Personally, I am highly disturbed, upset, and angry. Producers will even put a disclaimer at the start of the Image to indicate that there will be upsetting and graphic footage. If we were like lions, then these images would make us feel hungry, not upset.

Parents want to protect their children from watching upsetting content, especially when it is one of their favourite animals on the chopping block. Lions teach their cubs how to hunt and kill at a very young age. We try to create a disconnect and instead of telling our children that they are having cow stew for dinner, we will tell them that they are eating beef.

In closing, you could ask the person who made this excuse: "Now that we have established that we are not like other animals, how can we justify acting like them?"

EATING ANIMALS IS PART OF THE FOOD CHAIN

The food chain is not to be confused with the food pyramid that we are given when we go to a nutritionist or when following a diet. The food chain is a process that is important for the environment and ecosystem to maintain a healthy balance of plant and animal life. Without the natural food chain, we would have animal and plant species overpopulating the earth.

Instead of allowing nature to do what it has been doing since the beginning of time, humans have changed the course of the food chain. Plants need energy to grow, move, reproduce and survive. The food chain is a representation of how energy is passed between living things. An example simply explained is that the energy is passed from the sun to the grass, allowing it to grow. An insect gets its energy by eating the grass. A larger insect comes along and eats the smaller one and thus absorbs its energy. A bird flies overhead, sees the insect, and feeds on it, absorbing its energy.

The person you are talking to is right, animals are part of the natural food chain. However, humans have broken the natural order cycle of the food chain by deciding which animals they want to breed. The animals are then genetically modified and artificially inseminated to produce animals according to personal needs, wants, and desires.

Once the animals have reached their desired growth and weight, they are carted off to the slaughterhouses where they are hung upside down. Their throats are slashed or they are suffocated in gas chambers. Nothing about the factory farming industry is remotely comparable to the natural food chain. In fact, to state that "this is nature" is so far from the truth because the natural order of the food chain has nothing to do with the circumstances surrounding the processes involved.

Human beings are said to be at the top of the food chain because we eat both plants and animals. Just because we 'pride' ourselves on being at the top of the food chain does not morally justify us to dominate and exploit all living beings.

Yes, animals kill other animals to survive but as humans, we do not need to kill animals to survive. The food industry has progressed in such a way that animals are not needed to be eaten for survival as it may have been in our ancestral times.

If the person you are talking to states that eating animals is all part of the food chain, you could ask them to explain what the food chain looks like in nature. Ask them to explain what they believe is natural about the food chain that we have created in the animal agriculture industry.

To end off the conversation, leave your opponent with the following question: "Now that you know that animal agriculture is as far away from a natural food chain as possible, why would you continue contributing towards animal abuse when instead you could be kind and compassionate?"

I LOVE ANIMALS, BUT I ALSO LOVE MEAT

Nearly everyone you speak to will tell you that they love animals. There are billions of people walking on this earth that are pet owners. They are the loudest voices when advocating against the abuse of animals, whether it is organized dog fighting, hunting wildlife for trophies and entertainment purposes, or even telling your neighbours off for letting their dogs sleep outside. They participate in fundraisers for animal shelters and often will donate to animal causes.

All these actions would describe someone who claims to care a great deal about animals, but then every day they are drinking milk in their tea or coffee, eating some form of meat for their dinner, or eating that thick slice of chocolate cake made with milk and eggs. These are the people who are paying for the animals on the factory farms to be abused and slaughtered daily.

These people may love their pets, but they cannot say that they love animals. When you love something, you take care of it. You make sure it is happy and healthy. You do not want it to get hurt or injured. You definitely would not want it to die.

If the question is: "Can you love animals and also eat them?" I would say that the answer would be pretty simple: "No!"

What we may consider as pets in the United States, the United Kingdom, or Western countries, may be considered food in other parts of the world.

Dog Meat Festival

Yes, you are reading correctly. Since 2009, in the Chinese province of Yulin, Guangxi, the locals have hosted a lychee and dog meat festival. The annual event is held during the summer solstice and spans over a period of 10 days in June. This event has been criticized by animal cruelty organizations both locally and internationally.

The festival organizers have indicated that the thousands of dogs that are used for this festival are killed "humanely" and many have argued that eating dog meat is no different than eating the meat of any other animal. Animal activists, however, have been advocating against the cruelty by indicating that the dogs are tortured and boiled alive to enhance the flavour of the meat. There are also reports that of the thousands of dogs that have been used for this festival have been stolen from family homes in nearby villages.

Human beings live by double standards. They will advocate against dogs being killed and eaten for a summer solstice festival, but when it comes to slaughtering a pig, a cow, a sheep, or a chicken, they have no problem enjoying the meat. Sadly, people do not connect that the piece of meat on their plate was a living being. If humans had to slaughter animals themselves, I do believe that most of the people on the earth would be either vegetarian or vegan. All living creatures, regardless of whether they are pets or domestic animals, should have equal rights. They should all be allowed the right to be free and live their life without pain and fear.

A question you could ask the person you are talking to is: "Can you really say that you love all animals if you are willing to pay for them to be abused and killed?"

A Get-Together with Friends

I met up with Stacey and Belinda the other day. We were having a cup of coffee at the local coffee shop and I was telling them about an article I had read. The article went along the lines of how some foreign country was breeding cats for cat milk. I was telling them how they forcefully impregnate the cats, and once they have their kittens, the babies are taken away from their mothers. The purpose of this is so that the mother cats can be used for their milk.

Well, the look on Stacey and Belinda's faces was that of shock, horror, and disbelief.

"How disgusting!" They responded in unison.
"I cannot believe people would do something so cruel to cats!" Belinda said.

"Oh sorry, did I say cats?" I responded calmly, "I meant to say cows."

OUR ANCESTORS WERE MEAT EATERS

It is believed that humans evolved from the primate family. As you know, primates are apes, gorillas, and orangutans. They ate a plant-based diet that consisted of nuts, fruit, leaves, and some insects every now and again. Over time, the insects were replaced by raw, uncooked meat. As our ancestors evolved, so their intelligence levels changed. Their diets changed. No one is sure when they discovered fire and how they realized that they could cook their meat, but that is when their diets changed.

Time moves on, circumstances change, and history is where it is supposed to be–in the past. We should not be basing our current existence on what our ancestors did or did not do. The consumption of meat might have been a necessity during the famine and in times of food scarcity. Jumping into the present, we do not need to consume animal-based products because there is enough food being produced to feed the ever-expanding population. The necessity to eat meat is based on our preferences. By continuing to consume meat, eggs, and dairy, we are allowing our ancestors to guide us to the great beyond. Stop giving them the power to dictate our future.

You could ask the person you are talking to: "If your ancestors walked around in animal hides, why are you not following their example and doing the same today?"

If your opponent wants to argue that because our ancestors did it, we can do it too, then they need to follow in their footsteps. That will mean that we would have to sleep outside, get rid of our devices, and say goodbye to the modern comforts such as having a hot shower, a soft bed, using a toilet, and dressing in our name-branded clothing. The argument is unfounded because as man has evolved, so did the world. What worked for our ancestors will not be applicable to the modern world we live in.

Our ancestors were responsible for a large number of immoral acts against humans and animals. The acts they committed might have been acceptable in their time, but acts such as murder, slavery, and the sexual abuse of another human being are now a crime punishable by law. Unfortunately, the heinous acts such as force being used to impregnate a cow, the unnecessary murder of wildlife for trophies, forcing them to take drugs against their will, and the murder of innocent animals are overlooked and ignored because non-vegans deem it to be a worthy cause which was instigated by our ancestors. Yet knowing what they did, many still hold onto the belief that our ancestors gave us a purpose in life.

Something you could ask your opponent is: "Do you think we should base our values and morality on those of our primitive ancestors?"

"Do you believe that just because we have done something for centuries, that makes it acceptable in this day and age?"

EATING MEAT AND DAIRY IS PART OF MY TRADITION AND CULTURE

People may argue that they have to eat meat and animal products because it is part of their tradition or culture. You might hear people say: "How can we have a Thanksgiving feast without a turkey? It is tradition!"

Over the last 200 years, we have had many terrible traditions. One hundred and fifty years ago, slavery was a terrible tradition. One hundred years ago, women were not allowed to vote. Fifty years ago, African Americans were not treated as equals under the law. Twenty-five years ago, there were no rights for homosexuals. People have come to realize that traditions and cultures can be wrong and not morally justifiable.

You could ask the person you are talking to: "If slavery was a tradition, do you believe we should continue with this practice because it is traditional?"

Thankfully traditions and laws were changed because they were morally wrong.

What is happening to animals is no different than what happened to the slaves, the women that could not vote, the equal rights of all African Americans, or people who choose to love someone of the same sex. If people can have rights, so can animals. I live in hope that in the near future, a law will be passed that will ban animal slavery.

"Just because something is traditional is no reason to do it, of course."

— LEMONY SNICKET

Sadly, there are still many cruel traditions taking place throughout the world. We will explore these traditions and cultures.

Taiji Dolphin Hunt

Dolphins are one of the most beautiful sea mammals to grace the oceans around the world. Most of us know dolphins by visiting aquariums, watching television shows, or nature documentaries. These beautiful creatures are loving animals that enjoy frolicking in the ocean and if you are lucky enough to be a spectator on a cruise ship, you can see them leaping out of the water with grace as they entertain their audience.

Culture, as well as greed, was born in the coastal town of Taiji in Japan. Since 2010, Japanese fishermen have been participating in what is called the Taiji dolphin hunt. This event takes place from September to March. Every year, the fishermen force pods of dolphins into the bay of the coastal town. A handful of the dolphins are chosen and sold off to facilities such as aquariums, water parks, or hotels where they are held captive and trained to entertain visitors.

The dolphins that are not sold off, are herded into a cove where they are brutally killed and slaughtered with harpoons for their flesh. The blue water turns red following the massacre of hundreds of innocent dolphins, all because of greed.

Toro de la Vega

The Spanish town of Tordesillas has been hosting the traditional and cultural medieval bull festival since 1524. A lone bull, bewildered and feeling threatened is chased by hundreds of people on foot or on horseback, through the town. The mob of people are armed with lances which is a long wooden stick with a steel tip that they use to chase the bull away from the town where they then spear him to death.

Although the age-old tradition of killing the bulls has been banned since 2019, the annual festival-goers have continued chasing the bulls through the town, still traumatizing them.

Kots Kaal Pato

Every April, for more than 100 years, the Kots Kaal Pato was both a tradition and part of the culture of Mexicans who believed that the Yucatan ritual would bring rain. This cruel ritual saw small live animals strung up like pinatas and beaten to death or having their heads cut off. Thanks to various animal anti-cruelty organizations, the Kots Kaal Pato ritual was banned in 2016.

I get that culture is important to people from all walks of life but it does not mean that it is morally right. If you were to do some independent research, you will stumble across hundreds, if not thousands of cultural practices that are being practiced throughout the world. Not all cultural practices involve animals, but human beings as well.

In some countries, it is both culture and tradition for older men to take girls as young as 12 years of age, as their wives. There are young girls whose genitalia are mutilated because it is part of the culture, and to prevent them from having premarital sex. These cultural and traditional practices should not be taking place in present times.

Ask the person you are talking to: "Can you honestly say that we should base our morality on these cultural and traditional practices?"

Take a step back and think about what traditions and cultures say about people in present times. Christmas and Easter are perfect examples of tradition and culture. For these two holidays, everyone flocks to church for the services because that is how they were raised. For most, those are the only two occasions where they go to church other than the occasional wedding or funeral. Exchanging gifts and passing out Easter eggs is a tradition that is believed to have begun in the 1800s.

There are many more traditions that we can build and expand on such as dancing, singing, writing, or planting trees. What is stopping us from creating a unique tradition with friends and family that is special and adds honour and value to our future generations?

In closing you could ask your opponent: "Do you not believe that we should be focusing on these beautiful traditions instead and forget brutal and violent ones?"

THE FOCUS SHOULD BE ON HUMAN RIGHTS

No one is going to argue with you that our basic human rights are important. The right to have a warm bed to sleep in, decent food, medical care, respect, dignity, equality, and independence are part and parcel of our basic human rights. Unfortunately, not everyone is lucky enough to have those basic human rights because of unforeseen circumstances.

When I started on my vegan journey, I came across many people who have told me that I should not be wasting my energy on the rights of animals. I was told that if I want to make a difference, I should be focusing on human rights issues. I have seen homeless people as I walked through the streets of London and I have seen images of malnourished children when I turn on the television. I have also seen the fundraising campaigns that collect money and the various organizations that reach out to these people. I am not going to argue that these issues are not important, especially when the world is reeling due to a pandemic that has crippled the economy. No matter what you say or do, someone else will add their pennies to the pot with something that is more important.

Personally, I want to do something that means something and is important to me and know that I made a difference. I can give money to any of the organizations that are collecting for malnourished children, or donations towards cancer research, but how do I know that my money is going directly to these causes? I could resign from my job, fly to Africa and help build houses. I could even volunteer my free time to help at homeless shelters or feed the hungry at soup kitchens. All these options are time-consuming, costly, or inconvenient.

By embarking on my vegan journey, I knew that I would be doing something meaningful. Being a vegan has a huge impact, not just for animals, but also for the environment and people. It is something I can do with very little effort. It does not take up extra time and it is not going to cost me anything. I can carry on living my life the way I did before, with the added benefit of knowing that I am doing what I can for animals, the environment, and the people of the world.

People are not interested in focusing on the broader picture. They see what is in front of them, meaning they see images on the television and in printed media. They see and hear what they want and if it was not mentioned, it does not matter or affect them. In horse-racing circles, this is known as "wearing blinkers"–what you do not see cannot change your view.

The person you are talking to cares about human rights, but let us take a closer look at the fine print that is not mentioned on the packaging of the meat products, or any of the products found in our stores. Hopefully, this will put things into perspective and they will be able to lose the blinkers and see things through a clearer vision.

With a global population of over 7 billion people, it is estimated that approximately 925 million people are suffering from hunger, approximately 870 million people are suffering from malnutrition, and approximately 2.5 million children under the age of five, die yearly due to starvation. Underdeveloped and poor countries such as Africa and Asia are the most affected (World Animal Foundation, 2021).

Allow the person you are talking to the chance to think about the figures you presented them with, and then give them some more information. Growing crops of soybean and corn amount to millions of tons. Unfortunately, the millions of tons of grains do not make it onto the shelves in stores or pantries in our homes, as the majority of the crops are fed to the animals that are raised for consumption. Broken down, approximately 40% to 50% of the corn and 80% of the soybeans go directly to animal farming. It might not seem that significant to many people, but in a world where hunger, starvation, and malnutrition are rife, those crops could be used to feed those in need.

Instead of providing the necessary nourishment to those who need it most, the majority of the crops are used to feed the livestock. Yes, the animals need food to survive, but animal farming focuses on fattening up the livestock so that they can head off to the slaughterhouses, into the stores, and onto plates. Approximately 13 to 20 pounds of grain is used to build a cow's muscle mass by one pound, seven pounds of grain for one pound of pork, and four and a half pounds of grain for one pound of chicken. By not eating animal products anymore, you could potentially be feeding 13 to 20 times more people with the grains.

Many will claim that they want to help people. Remind your opponent that they have no problem eating animal products knowing how much food is being wasted to provide non-vegans with a piece of meat. Surely this is a humanitarian issue. If people are fighting for the basic human rights of others, then they should be made aware of just how wrong they are.

It is time for every person to have their voices heard. It is our human right to be heard, and it is our human right to express our feelings. There are millions of people that are forced to take on jobs to provide for their families. Many of these jobs exploit their workers and infringe on their human rights. When people are desperate to do the right thing, such as earning an income, nobody seems to care as long as they are off the streets, not committing crimes, and not begging.

Slaughter houses

An anonymous source spoke to the British Broadcasting Corporation (BBC) about his experience working in a slaughterhouse. He starts off by telling the interviewer that as a child, he has always wanted to be a veterinarian. Sadly, it was a dream that never materialized and he ended up working in a slaughterhouse for six years. His job was that of the quality controller and his job was to ensure that the quota of approximately 250 cows a day was killed.

No matter what anyone says, a slaughterhouse is a sad and dirty place. The floors are covered with animal feces and guts, and the walls are covered in blood. He recalls the smells as he enters the building. It was as if an invisible person was suffocating him as he inhaled the smell of dying animals.

He recalls that the cows that were brought in to be slaughtered were scared and panicked. The cows would be stunned before being hoisted to the machine that would slaughter them, and many times the cows would spasm and kick the workers. The guilt that he and his co-workers felt was real and terrifying. He never experienced any of the physical injuries, but it did affect his mind. He was plagued by nightmares as he remembered his day at work, and the horrors he had witnessed (BBC, January 2020).

Ask the person you are talking to how their mental health would be affected, if they had to go to work each day and kill hundreds of animals that never hurt them.

Destruction of Tropical Forests

We have touched on the effects that deforestation poses to the environment, but some effects infringe on the human rights of millions of indigenous and traditional people who have been living in the Amazon Basin for centuries. With the global population on the increase yearly, the demand for animal agriculture increases, and with that, so does the need for expansion.

Cattle farming in Brazil's Amazon is responsible for the illegal seizing of land, thus forcing communities to find accommodation elsewhere. The farmers bulldoze, burn and chop the trees to create clear areas for the cattle to graze, as well as grow crops to feed them. Thanks to the destruction of the forests, the indigenous people who still live in the area are being plagued with fires destroying what is left of their land and homes.

Tanneries

The leather shoes, wallets, purses, and jackets non-vegans like using pose one of the biggest human rights issues in the world. Third-world countries such as Bangladesh and India employ the services of adults and approximately 8,000 to 12,000 children under the age of 17. These people, who are willing to work up to 14 hours a day, seven days a week are being paid less than $2.00 per day (Admin, 2016).

Working for next to nothing, with the amount of hours they put in each day, is nothing in comparison to the unsafe conditions they are exposed to. These workers are exposed to harmful chemicals which are used to make those leather products many people cannot live without. Their working conditions are terrible as they are placed in a room that has very little ventilation and are required to stomp on animal hides in tubs of toxic chemicals.

The workers suffer from all types of health problems. Short-term problems include aching bodies, acid burns and rashes, chest problems, light-headedness, nausea, and vision problems. If these short-term health problems do not shock your opponent, then ask them how they would feel if it was their children, nieces, nephews, or neighbour's children suffering from these conditions. Long-term health problems are far more severe and include different types of cancers, disfiguration, amputation, skin diseases, and death. It is believed that the children who work in these tanneries have a life expectancy of up to 50 years–if they are lucky (Biswas & Rahman, 2013).

After reading about the exploitation of workers who work and live in sectors that involve animal agriculture, you have a clearer understanding of my choice to be a vegan, and why I am passionate about saving animals. Just because I adopted the vegan lifestyle, does not make me care less about my fellow human beings who are being traumatized, driven from their homes, or maimed. It makes me care even more, because if we all stopped eating meat, every exploited person would have a chance at a better life. A new direction in the job market would be created for millions that would not involve putting their mental and physical health at risk.

In closing, ask the person you are talking to: "How do you think we can justify feeding 56 billion land animals every year, but cannot feed 800 million women, men, and children who are suffering and dying of starvation?"

I NEED TO EAT MEAT AND DAIRY TO BE HEALTHY

This is a common excuse that non-vegans throw into every argument when they hear that you are following the vegan lifestyle. People are looking for excuses to justify the fact that they need dairy, eggs, and animal flesh for health reasons, and ignore the processes involved in getting those products to our tables.

Yes, it is true that our bodies need vitamins and nutrients to stay healthy. By following a plant-based diet, we will get all the necessary vitamins and nutrients our bodies need without having to put the life of an animal at risk. There are so many misconceptions surrounding the vegan lifestyle, that those who are uninformed will believe anything that is told to them. It is possible to live a long and healthy life by following the vegan lifestyle.

Your opponent will tell you that if you do not consume animal products, you will be putting your health at risk. However, as you know, this is not true.

According to research done by the largest nutrition and diet professionals in Britain and the United States of America, if you are following a plant-based diet correctly, you can get all the necessary protein, vitamins, and minerals your body needs. Pregnant and lactating women can get the essential nutrients that are needed to be healthy. Babies and children can follow a vegan diet and still get all the nutrients that are necessary to promote growth without compromising their health (McManus, 2018).

Protein

Our bodies need protein. That is a fact. Our skin, muscles, bones, and organs need the essential amino acids to be healthy. Meat and dairy provide those essential amino acids, but you can also get them by eating a plant-based diet.

- Grains
- Legumes and pulses
- Nuts and seeds
- Tofu
- Soymilk
- Fruit and vegetables

Iron

Iron helps to produce red blood cells which carry the oxygen through your body. In order to help your body absorb iron, you should include vitamin C in your diet.

- Lentils, beans and chickpeas
- Nuts and seeds
- Dried fruit such as apricots and raisins.
- Rice, wheat, oats and quinoa
- Dark leafy greens

Calcium

This is one that has everyone convinced they need to consume dairy. Calcium is essential to our health. If we do not get sufficient calcium in our diets, we face a diagnosis of osteoporosis which weakens our bones that can cause breaks or loss of our teeth.

- Soybeans
- Green leafy vegetables, such as kale, broccoli and spinach
- Sesame seeds and tahini
- White and brown bread
- Fortified plant milk
- Breakfast cereal

Vitamin B12

Iron and Vitamin B12 fall into the same category in that their addition to our diet helps produce red blood cells. Vitamin B12 is found in fish, meat, and dairy products. However, vitamin B12 is not something that is naturally found in animal flesh. Vitamin B12 is something that is found in the dirt/earth. The animals get their vitamin B12 by eating dirt. In the case of factory farming, the animals do not live in fields and meadows, so they cannot ingest vitamin B12 by eating dirt with the grass, so they are injected or their food is fortified with the necessary vitamins such as vitamin B12. In fact, approximately 95% of vitamin B12 supplements that are being manufactured are given to farm animals.

If we were out hiking or walking through the meadows and pulled a carrot out of the ground, dusted off the dirt, and ate it, we would naturally be ingesting vitamin B12. Because we buy our fruit and vegetables in supermarkets, we do not get the essential vitamin B12. Luckily, most vegan alternatives are fortified with vitamin B12.

- Plant-based milk
- Nutritional yeast
- Breakfast cereal
- Yeast extracts such as Marmite and Vegemite

Something you could ask the person you are talking to is: "Where do you think animals get their protein and nutrients from?"

Elephants and rhinos are two of the largest land animals in the world. Their diets consist of plant-based sources. They are classed as herbivores. Herbivores do not eat any meat and live off plants and plant matter. If you have ever seen an elephant or a rhino, you might notice that they are not small animals. Their diet suggests that they do not need anything else to supplement their meals.

Herbivorous animals such as cows and sheep get their protein by eating grass and plant matter, so they are getting "first-hand" protein. By following the vegan lifestyle, we are getting our protein source "first-hand" from plant-based foods. On the other hand, when humans eat meat, they are consuming processed "second-hand" protein. Believe it or not, meat protein is not as good for our bodies as plant protein is.

As mentioned previously, consuming animal products is linked to an array of illnesses. The American Cancer Society, with the backing of the International Agency for Research on Cancer (IARC), has classified processed meat as a type 1 carcinogen, meaning it is linked to causing various types of cancer (IARC, 2018).

A carcinogen, according to the Merriam-Webster dictionary, is a substance or agent that can potentially cause cancer in living tissue. Eating processed meat, smoking, and inhaling asbestos are classed as carcinogenic. Shockingly, this all translates back to the fact that eating processed meats is just as likely to cause cancer as smoking.

A documentary worth watching is The Game Changers on Netflix. This show was directed by Louie Psihoyos, along with executive producers James Cameron, Jackie Chan, Novak Djokovic, Chris Paul, Arnold Schwarzenegger, and Lewis Hamilton, and released in 2018. The documentary follows James Wilks as he travels around the world to learn about nutrition and what would be the optimal diet for his recovery after an injury.

After meeting with researchers in Austria, he realized that he, just like many of our meat-eating friends, was under the impression that we need animal protein to build muscle. The Austrian researchers educated him that the Roman gladiators trained and competed by following a vegan lifestyle. James, who is a combative instructor for the United States Military and was a former UFC fighter until his injury (The Game Changers, 2018).

Other famous sporting heroes include:

- Fiona Oakes, who holds four world records for marathon running.
- Patrik Baboumian, strongman competitor with several world records.
- Kyrie Irving, who is a professional basketball player in the NBA.
- Colin Kaepernick, former professional football quarterback.
- Kendrick Farris, Olympic weightlifter from the United States.

These are men and women who are and have been competing in sport while actively following a vegan diet. We can get all the nutrients, minerals, and vitamins we need from plants to live a long, happy, and healthy life.

In conclusion, ask the person you are talking to: "Now that you know that we can get all our nutrients from plants, can we still justify abusing and killing animals if it is not necessary?"

IT IS MY PERSONAL CHOICE

When people discover that you are vegan, they become defensive. The most common statements I hear are: "It is my personal choice, respect the way I do things" or "stop pushing your views on others."

If I have to be honest with you, these are statements I also used before I adopted the vegan lifestyle. Just because we have our own personal choices does not mean that they are justified. When someone's "personal choice" impacts the lives of others, is it still a personal choice?

We all live in the same world, and we watch the news and hear stories about what is going on in other countries. People are more concerned about lives that are lost to nonsensical crimes, fighting, poverty, drought, or starvation. No one really takes notice that the world we claim to love so much is being destroyed by animal agriculture. When people support the industry which is destroying the world I live in, then their personal choice is affecting my life too.

Imagine that you are taking a stroll along the beach, lapping up the beauty as the seagulls dive into the water to snatch up a fish, or as they playfully chase each other around on the sand. In the distance you see a couple having a romantic picnic. As you get closer, you notice that they are packing up. They fold up their blanket and pick up their picnic basket and start walking away. You notice that they have left their plastic cutlery, containers, wrappers, and bottles behind.

You could ask the person you are talking to: "Just because a person has a personal choice, does that make it okay for them to do whatever they want? Is it okay to leave all the trash on the beach just because it was their personal choice?"

In 2018, an impatient driver put his personal choice above his morals. As he came to a stop at the traffic lights in the CBD of Cape Town, in South Africa, a family of Egyptian geese and their six goslings were crossing the road. Ironically, it was a pedestrian crossing and if you know the rules of the road, if you enter the crossing, you have the right of way. The traffic light had changed and despite people flagging him down to prevent him from driving, the driver ignored everyone and intentionally drove over the goslings. Witnesses at the scene were distraught as the mother goose cried for the loss of two of her children.

In May of 2020, three men made a choice to ignore lockdown restrictions and to go to Hardwick Park in County Durham in the United Kingdom. At the park, these three men, armed with sticks, started attacking ducks for no apparent reason. Members of the community who witnessed the attack from their homes contacted the police who were dispatched to the park. One of the men was arrested at the park, and the other two were later caught after a search. One of the mallard ducks was killed and the second one was taken to the vet where they hoped he would recover from his injuries.

These senseless acts of injury and murder to innocent animals cannot be justified by saying it was a personal choice. What kind of person does it take to wake up one morning and decide that today is a good day to plough through a flock of geese or go to a park and intentionally kill ducks for pleasure?

Unfortunately, animals can't inform us of their personal choices, because they do not have a voice to tell us what they would like. We do know that they live in fear, not knowing what tomorrow or the next day will bring or whether they will live to see another day. Vegans and organizations such as Anonymous for the Voiceless are using their voices to fight for the land and marine animals every day. Every year over 56 billion land animals and 2.7 trillion marine animals are slaughtered. (Green, 2016)

Ask the person you are talking to: "What about the personal choice of the animals?"

Billions of animal lives are sacrificed every year to make clothing and accessories. The skin of the animals is used to make leather products, the feathers of ducks and geese are used to fill pillows or duvets, and some small animals such as foxes and rabbits, are kept in cages until they are killed for their fur. Goats and sheep are beaten and mutilated for their wool, cashmere, and mohair.

Thousands of animals are not allowed to have the freedom to do what comes naturally to them. Elephants, bears, monkeys, and horses are trained to perform tricks at the circus. These animals have no choice but to keep up with their training, as they are punished if they do not perform as expected. As if harming them during training is not bad enough, think about the method of transport to get from one show to the next. They are forced into semi-truck trailers, they are kept in chains, they have no natural bedding in their cages, their cages are often dirty, and they are separated from their families. Many of these animals are forced to entertain people until the day they die.

Thinking about the different medications, vaccines and medical treatments, the makeup we wear, and even the body lotions we use all have to be tested before they can be distributed to the public. All across the world, in research facilities and laboratories, you will find mice, rats, cats, dogs, monkeys, and other types of animals living in cages. These defenceless animals are living in fear while waiting for the next dose of medication or procedure to be performed on them.

End the conversation by asking the person you are talking to if just because someone has a personal choice, does that make it morally justifiable?

I COULD NEVER GIVE UP ANIMAL PRODUCTS BECAUSE I LIKE THE TASTE

No one is going to argue that meat and dairy products taste good. Believe it or not, vegans ate meat and animal products as well and they enjoyed it. Vegans do not stop eating animal products because they do not like the taste, it is because of a realization that we were enjoying something that once had a mother and a father. It was a connection that clicked on a personal level that made us decide to give up eating and using animal-based products.

When meat-eaters are biting into that piece of steak, no one thinks about where that steak came from. The labels on the packaging may tell us that the animals were raised as organic and free-grazing, but that is as far as it goes. If we visit farms, we see the cows and their calves and we get given a bag of grain to treat them with. After the visit, we go home and we think nothing of what their future is going to be like.

The reality of the matter is that those calves are taken away from their mothers, so we can have their milk. Cows like humans carry their babies for nine months. When the calf gets taken from the mother, the mother will look for her calf and cry out for it. I have seen heart-breaking videos of cows running after the trucks, trying to get their babies back. These animals form close bonds, just like humans.

The mother cow will experience this traumatizing procedure multiple times in her life until she can no longer produce the milk that is required. Then she gets sent off to the slaughterhouse where she is hung upside down, her throat slit and dismembered to provide non-vegans with meat for their dinner. What happens to the calves? If they are female they are raised to take their mother's position of producing offspring and continuing the cycle. If they are male, they are usually deemed as a waste product and are killed. In some cases, they will get slaughtered for veal.

Most people, when confronted with the imagery you are explaining, will not believe you because it is easier to ignore when you have not seen something first-hand. On some level, the person you are talking to may believe what you are saying, but it is easier to be in denial or dismiss it as happening elsewhere in some third-world countries because they choose to believe that first-world countries do not practice such cruelty.

Here are some documentaries you could advise people to watch, depending on which country they are from:

- A land of hope and Glory: This shows undercover footage of factory farms in the United Kingdom
- Earthlings: This is mixed footage throughout the globe, predominantly in the United States
- Dominion: This is undercover footage of factory farming in Australia

Ask the person you are talking to if they value their taste buds higher than the life of an animal. Most of the people you come across will say no. You could ask them why they would compromise their morals by eating the flesh of animals who were once living, breathing creatures who harmed no one and did not ask to become food.

If they tell you that their taste buds mean more to them than the life of an animal or that they do not care, you could ask them to explain why they value their taste over an animal's life. In many cases, this will lead to more excuses such as needing to eat meat for protein.

After reading through everything that has previously been mentioned thus far, you have more than enough arguments to help them see the truth.

Just because we enjoy something does not mean that it is morally right or that it is the right thing to do. If we think about the mother cow that we mentioned. She goes through the whole cycle of being pregnant, giving birth, nurturing her calf until it is forcefully removed from her so that she can provide us with milk. She is being used and abused over and over again so that we can have our favourite cheese, double-thick milkshakes, creamy ice creams, and all other types of milk-based products. After all her 'service' of bearing calves and being milked, she is not sent to the pasture to retire and live her life in peace and harmony–no, she is taken to the slaughterhouse to become food.

Considering the processes involved in breeding and raising animals for consumption, the farm-to-table scenario can take months, or even years to provide us with meat for our meals. How long does it take to cook a piece of steak, a pork chop, or a piece of fish? On average, you are looking at spending between 10 and 20 minutes preparing a meal that will take even less time to consume. This meal will cost an animal its life.

Ask the person who used this excuse: "Do you think it is acceptable to inflict violence, pain, and suffering on animals so that we can satisfy our taste buds?"

One thing that non-vegan people are most concerned about is that they believe they will only be eating fruit and vegetables. Over the last 20 years or so, the vegan food market has evolved and come up with innovative plant-based alternatives that replicate meat products. Stores and supermarkets have dedicated sections that cater to the needs of vegans. Fast food restaurants have joined the vegan party and offer alternatives so that everyone can enjoy their favourites.

Stores such as Walmart in the United States, and Tesco in the United Kingdom, and many other stores all over the world offer a variety of vegan meals and milk alternatives. If you were under the impression that you would be eating boring and bland food, you are about to discover that boring and bland do not feature in the vegan way of life.

- Plant-based breakfast sausage that is free of meat, gluten, soy, and GMO
- A plant-based mayonnaise that is free of eggs
- Chicken nuggets that are free of chicken
- Vegan mac and cheese
- Vegan chocolate chip cookies
- Plant-based chipotle chick'n power bowls
- Burger patties that taste like meat, but are 100% plant-based
- Breaded chicken wings without the chicken and made with cauliflower
- Vegan cheese without dairy
- Chocolate milk puddings made with almond milk, which is free of soy, dairy, and gluten
- Vegan egg made from plants
- Avocado oil butter
- Vegan ice cream

The list of vegan-friendly foods is endless, and you are guaranteed to enjoy guilt-free meals knowing that you are saving animals. The best news of all is that your taste buds will not be able to tell the difference between the meat it has been eating for years or the plant-based food. It is a case of mind over matter, and a simple change such as eliminating animal products from your diet is the first step in the morally right direction.

IF WE DO NOT EAT THEM, WE WOULD HAVE TOO MANY ANIMALS

Another popular excuse is that if everyone in the world decided to stop eating meat, dairy, and eggs, the world would be overrun with cows, pigs, and chickens. As much as we would love for everyone to go vegan overnight, it is an unrealistic expectation.

Realistically, if everyone were to become vegan over time, the change would be gradual. By the time the entire population became fully vegan, there would not be as many animals left. There would be a decline in the number of animals being bred, so the concern about farm animals overrunning the world would not be a problem.

Consumers are made up of people who earn or have money. We take our money to the stores or go online and we buy what we need. Our preferences and needs determine what we buy and this, in turn, alerts the suppliers who keep producing based on what we purchase.

Animal agriculture is no different than any other industry. The more meat and dairy we buy, the more animals are needed to fulfil the demand. Farmers will continue breeding animals based on our demands. If everyone stopped eating meat, drinking milk, and using eggs all at once, it would cripple the animal agriculture industry. Of course, if there was a gradual decrease in the demand for animal products, the prices would increase making it expensive to purchase.

The effects on the supply and demand during the global pandemic are indicative of what the economic impact would be on animal agriculture. Across the world, hundreds of thousands of laborers tested positive for the coronavirus. As per the requirements of the World Health Organization (WHO) and many other health organizations, everyone that tested positive needed to be quarantined for up to two weeks and if there were any implications, even longer. Although the demand was still high, the supply had decreased and the prices increased to make up for it.

Some people may ask you if farm animals could face extinction if everyone became vegan.

Farm animals fall under the category of domesticated animals that have been bred, genetically modified, and adapted to provide us with food. This process has been happening for thousands of years. These animals were chosen because of certain traits:

- They grow quickly
- They mature quicker
- They are easy to breed in captivity
- They are herbivores and cost-efficient to feed
- They adapt to the conditions in which they are in
- They are herd animals that are easier to control

Looking at the traits, you will understand why a dairy cow could produce up to ten times more milk in captivity than what is normal. Chickens have been genetically modified to grow bigger in a short amount of time.

In answer to their question, it is very possible that farm animals could face extinction as they would not be relying on humans for care. We would be restoring the natural ebb and flow of the food chain. One might argue that this is as unethical as eating them, but if we allow nature to be restored, we would gain more natural biodiversity, which would save our planet for future generations.

Animal agriculture is responsible for the destruction of habitats and rainforests, the extinction of animal species, and ocean dead zones. Every second of every day, an acre of land is destroyed to make room for the meat industry. If we do not start changing how we eat and view the planet, we will run out of land to house an ever-growing population.

If we became vegan, we would eventually be saying goodbye to the cows that have given us milk and meat, and the chickens that have given us eggs and meat, but we would be saving millions of animal species that are being forced out of their natural habitats.

BUT PLANTS FEEL PAIN TOO

This is an excuse that many meat-eaters use as a line of defence when they face vegans. I dislike this excuse, as it tends to end in a heated argument. It feels as if they are trying to come up with any excuse to prove that they are right and that you do not know what you are talking about. When you are faced with someone that comes up with an excuse like this, or any similar excuse regarding plants, initiate a conversation without being annoyed.

Plants, unlike any other living and breathing creatures, do not have a central nervous system, pain receptors, or a brain. It is true that some plants have the ability to sense when insects crawl over them, or like the Venus flytrap that reacts to a flying insect and is able to trap its victim in approximately half a second. Plants are alive, they grow, eat and reproduce, but they cannot feel.

Humans and animals have the ability to walk away if they feel danger or pain. We can argue that we have evolved over time to do this or that God created us to feel the pain to protect us from our surroundings. However plants cannot walk away, if plants felt pain the way humans and animals do, why would they not have evolved over time to be able to escape. And if the person you are discussing this with believes that God created the world, then why would he be so cruel to create pain in plants and let them suffer so terribly without being able to defend themselves.

In truth, you cannot compare plucking a carrot from the ground or biting into an apple to the pain inflicted when cutting the throat of a cow to be slaughtered.

If the person you are talking to is still not satisfied with your reasoning, you could approach the argument from another direction. Start by explaining that in order to get one kilogram or 2.2 pounds of animal flesh, they need to consume up to 16 kilograms or 35 pounds of plants. The ratio is alarming when considering the difference between what is eaten and what is produced for human consumption. If the plants that are used to feed the animals were used to feed us directly, there would be more than enough food to feed the entire population. We would need to harvest fewer plants if we did not consume meat and dairy.

Something you could say to them is: "For the sake of the discussion, let us say that plants do feel pain, are you aware that a cow eats a lot more plants than a human, so vastly more plants are sacrificed for animal products than they are for vegan products?"

Continue the conversation by asking them what their thoughts are surrounding the destruction of the Amazon rainforest and the millions of trees being cut down to make room for animal agriculture. Surely, if plants feel pain, then the trees would be crying out in pain as well. Right about now would be an ideal opportunity to bring up that animals cry out in pain when they are being carted off to the slaughterhouse. These are sounds that are real and heart-wrenching. These are living animals that have brains, no matter the size, they have hearts and they feel pain.

ANIMALS DO NOT FEEL PAIN THE WAY HUMANS DO

Before you let the previous discussion frazzle out, keep the conversation going and present them with more information. The whole idea is to show them that what they believe to be right is not necessarily so. Restate your statement that animals have central nervous systems and that they can feel pain and emotions.

Most countries have animal cruelty laws in place for the protection of all animals. The abuse of animals ranges from neglect such as deprivation of food, water, shelter, or veterinary care to intentionally torturing, maiming, or murder. Even though there are laws, there are many loopholes that see offenders walking away with a slap on the wrist or a fine, and in extreme cases, a jail sentence and fine.

As with the animal cruelty laws, most countries have laws in place for the treatment of animals going to and while in the slaughterhouses. The Humane Slaughter Act was passed in 1958, which made it a law that animals at slaughterhouses be stunned until they are unconscious, secured, their throats cut and bled out before they can feel any pain. If you watch any of the documentaries that have been mentioned previously, you will notice that this does not always happen.

In addition, it was advised that inspectors from the United States Department of Agriculture (USDA) were to be present at slaughterhouses during the processes, as well as to inspect the area for cleanliness and to monitor diseases. A California slaughterhouse, which was the only USDA registered facility, was shut down after it was found that cattle had cancer. The USDA had to recall and dispose of 8.7 million pounds of already-processed meat (Linnekin, 2017)

I have heard the explanation of "humane slaughter" and this is one I do not agree with. It is believed that the animals are protected from pain, fear, and suffering when they are stunned into a state of shock or unconsciousness so that they cannot feel pain.

A question you could ask the person you are talking to is: "What do you understand by the word humane?"

Humane is another word for compassion. If your pet was sick and it was suffering a great deal, you would consider putting it down, because you have compassion for your pet and do not want it to suffer. I highly doubt anyone would send their pet to a slaughterhouse to stop its suffering.

Continue the conversation by asking them: "How can you humanely kill a healthy animal that does not want to die?"

It is an oxymoron to believe that you can humanely kill animals. You cannot humanely take the life of an animal, or person for that matter, that does not want to be killed. Those animals that are loaded up onto the trucks know what awaits them. They are afraid. They might only be animals, but they sense things more than most human beings, because it is in their nature.

If your opponent is still on the fence about whether animals feel pain, refer them to a study conducted by the British Veterinary Association in 2018. The article in question was written by Dr. Karina Bech Gleerup who researched pain management and the level of pain tolerance in horses. For any doctor to make a diagnosis in humans and animals, there are many procedures and tests that need to be performed which could be uncomfortable and painful. It is important to pinpoint the exact location of the pain and ascertain the damage before medication and treatment can commence.

To gauge the level of pain in a horse, Dr. Gleerup notes that owners will notice a change in the behaviour of the horse. Another tell-tale sign will be that the horse will want to be away from crowds or antisocial. It is pretty clear that horses, like humans, feel pain and want to be left alone, especially when they have colic or pulled a muscle (Gleerup, 2018).

In an article written by Karin Evans for the Greater Good Magazine, Ms. Evans writes about the Dutch primatologist, Frans de Waal. Mr. de Waal wrote a book, Mama's Last Hug: Animal Emotions and What They Tell Us about Ourselves (Evans, 2019). In the book, Mr. de Waal writes about an elderly biology professor by the name of Jan van Hooff who went to the Netherlands zoo to visit an elderly chimpanzee, Mama, who was in the last stages of her life. It is not recommended that humans enter enclosures for fear of violent attacks. Mr. van Hooff went into the enclosure and Mama reached out to him, hugged him, and patted his back. It is believed that she was letting him know that everything was okay.

After Mama passed away, Mr. de Waal looked on as the remaining chimpanzees in the enclosure paid their last respect to her. They were touching, washing, anointing, and cleaning her body as they mourned the loss of their beloved Mama (de Waal, 2019).

In conclusion, yes animals do feel pain. They have a central nervous system. If they had a voice and could speak out, they would be able to tell us where their pain is and how they really are feeling.

And yes, animals do feel emotional pain. As a human mother would mourn the loss of her baby, animals mourn the loss of their babies being forcefully removed from them. As you would mourn the loss of a partner, so your cat or dog would mourn the loss of his partner or his human companion.

Humans are at an advantage in both instances. If we feel pain, we can go to the doctor or we can take a painkiller from the medicine cabinet to ease the pain. If we suffer an emotional loss, we can speak to someone for comfort or join a support group. Why should animals suffer in silence?

ANIMALS SHOULD BE THANKFUL THAT WE ARE GIVING THEM LIFE

People seem to believe that we are doing animals a favour by breeding them into existence. We are using them for our pleasure and selfish needs such as entertainment, companionship, protection, or human consumption. If we were to apply the same logic to human situations, would we be saying that they are lucky to be alive?

Imagine that you are in a situation where one of your children or a member of your family has cancer or a disease that can be cured by someone in your family. The option of a donor is not up for discussion. The parents decide to have another baby, sometimes multiple babies if one does not have the required genes for that life-saving transplant or transfusion. These babies or children are referred to as "spare parts babies."

Having a baby should be one of the happiest days of your life. You have nine months to prepare for this little life. Like animals, you have an obligation to your baby to feed, nurture and protect it with your life. Unfortunately, some babies and children are not that lucky. If born into an abusive family, that little life will be neglected, starved, beaten, or sexually abused. The end result, in many cases, is death. Could we say that these children, as presented in the examples, should be thankful that they were conceived and given life?

If we look at pigs. Remembering the classic movies such as Charlotte's Web or Babe, we are led to believe that pigs roam freely and are happy all the time. In the world of factory farming, this is an illusion. When pigs are born, their tails are cut off and their teeth are clipped without any pain medication. They are put into small cages and as they grow, they are moved. Female pigs are used for breeding. They are kept in cages with no room to move or turn around, and bars separate them from their friends. She cannot escape from the two-by-one cage that is keeping her hostage. This proud pig is forced to sleep and eat in her feces, whereas in a natural setting, she would keep her 'bedroom', 'kitchen', and 'bathroom' separate. When the female pigs have reached their quotas of having babies, or if they become sick or old, they are carted off to the slaughterhouse.

Should these mommy pigs be grateful that they are being used as breeding machines, popping out babies they cannot bond with, living in a two-by-one cage, and be in pain from being cramped up day in and day out?

Nobody, humans or animals, should be 'grateful' to live a life of pain. How can this even be referred to as 'life'? Being born into a world or family that expects us to be thankful for the life we have been given when suffering abuse and torture is barely an existence.

End the conversation by asking: "Would you be grateful to live this kind of life?"

CAN'T WE JUST IMPROVE THE LIVES OF ANIMALS?

This is a suggestion that comes up quite often and has previously been discussed in multiple parts of this book. No matter how humanely animals are treated, they still end up being tortured and killed for the purpose of putting food on a plate, eggs in a cake, and milk in someone's tea. The packages of meat, poultry, eggs, and milk are labelled with various labels such as organic and free-range. Seeing these labels eases the guilt when buying their favourite animal products.

For the Sake of Free-Range

In my world, I like to believe that everyone cares about animals and that we really do not want them to suffer unnecessarily. Being a former meat-eater, I understand how non-vegans think and even though we mean well, we are just a little misguided. We tend to believe what health organizations and food regulators tell us. We even believe what the labels on the packages tell us.

When asking someone why they choose to buy free-range eggs, chicken or beef, you only have to hear their answers to know that they too believe what the labels tell them. If you think about free-range animals, you have a mental image of cows and sheep roaming around on millions of acres of luscious green pastures, and chickens running between them as they merrily peck at the ground. Sorry, but that mental image is about to become distorted. Free-range does not necessarily mean that the animals are roaming around the property or in pastures. If the animals are allowed in fenced-off areas, regardless of the size of the area, they are deemed to be free-range. The same applies to chickens. The space they are in does not have to be open. As long as they can have some fresh air and room to move, that is regarded as being free-range.

For the Sake of Organic

Whether growing produce or raising animals, farmers have to be certified as per the stipulations of the USDA. For example, the soil on the farm has to be free of prohibited substances such as harmful pesticides and synthetic fertilizers for at least three years. This includes grazing pastures and the feed for the animals. Once the organic certification has been awarded, the farms and the processes are subjected to yearly inspections by inspectors from the USDA. During these inspections, the soil is tested. Of concern as well is the health of the crops, the seeds being used, how weeds and pests are controlled, sufficient water systems and how contamination and potential risks are prevented.

On the meat side of the organic fence, regulations are clear that the animals are to receive better treatment than living in fenced enclosures with hardly any room to move. They are to be fed with 100% organic food, such as grains, grass and hay. No medications such as antibiotics or hormones to boost growth are permitted. They are allowed to be kept in a natural environment, such as living in pastures where they can graze freely.

Regardless of what the labels say or the images we see regarding free-range or organic, farmers still have to go through the process of fulfilling the supply and demand for consumers. The images we see make us believe that all is good on the factory farms. Seemingly happy animals grazing in luscious pastures are shown in advertisements, but it is only an image of their current conditions. I have never seen images on packages, labels or advertisements showing the animals being carted off to the slaughterhouse. I have never seen images of the look of terror in their eyes on any of the products in the stores.

In reality, there is not enough land to accommodate millions of grazing animals and this would have a greater impact on our environment. Even if the animals were allowed to roam freely, how could we morally justify removing them from their happy places to be slaughtered? After all, these animals that are allowed to roam and graze freely are having a "good life" before they become food.

"How can you humanely kill an animal that does not want to die?"

We have discussed the thought process of humane slaughter in a previous section, but it is worth bringing it up again for the sake of the discussion. If the person you are talking to still believes that animals are humanely slaughtered, ask them how they would 'compassionately' kill an animal that has been taken from its green pasture.

You could also try approaching the conversation from another angle and give them a human example.

"Imagine if you or a loved one was kidnapped. The kidnapper puts you in a beautifully decorated room that has a nice, warm and comfortable bed. He is making sure that you are comfortable in your new situation. He takes you outside for 10 minutes a day to have some fresh air. He feeds you three warm meals a day, makes you tea or coffee, and gives you biscuits or treats. At any time of the day or night, he comes to your room to abuse or rape you."

Ask some follow-up questions: "Have the improved living conditions for the victim made the situation any better? Would this be considered as 'humane' or 'ethical' kidnapping and abuse?"

At the end of the day, it is all good to say that the animals are free-range or organic, but those labels on the packaging reflect two opposite sides of the pole. In the end, most of it comes down to marketing. The labels are there to ease the meat eater's conscience. The animals do not care if they are labelled organic or their eggs free range.

Improving the living conditions of animals is not the answer. All animals want to be free, live a happy life without fear, pain and human exploitation.

MORALITY IS SUBJECTIVE

When we are born, we have instincts about what is right or wrong. A baby will know when it is hungry, unhappy, or has a wet or soiled diaper and they will let their parents or caregivers know. As the babies grow older, they are guided by their peers with an understanding of what is right or wrong. The words 'yes' or 'no' will be used to guide them. Our parents and caregivers can verbalize their intentions at a level that is appropriate for children to understand as they grow.

As adults, equipped with the dos and don'ts passed on from our parents, we are left to make decisions based on what we believe is right, wrong, moral or immoral. This is something that is ingrained in us, and it is up to us to make the right decisions. We know that drinking, smoking, or doing drugs is wrong, but people still do it. It might not fall into the clause of morality but for the sake of the argument, these are choices we choose to make.

Imagine a world where morality was subjective. We would not need the judges to determine our fate, lawyers to defend us, or police to arrest us, because there would be no differentiation between good and bad. No matter what we choose to do, our behaviour would be acceptable. We could steal to our heart's content or sexually assault and abuse adults and children without worrying about the consequences. Perhaps taking the life of innocent people would be 'okay'. Is this the kind of world we want to live in?

If you were to ask people if this was the kind of world they wanted to live in, I can assure you that 99% would say no. The remaining 1% would be those who choose to live a life of immorality and are not bothered by the rules of right and wrong.

Animals have a degree of morality. Although they cannot tell us that they are sorry for what they did, we can see it in their eyes and body language. If a dog makes a mess on your carpet by accident, you will reprimand him. His tails stop wagging, his ears droop, and he will look away from you. When he does look at you, you will see him make "puppy dog eyes" asking for your forgiveness. If you were to visit a factory farm on the day that the animals are being loaded up into trucks to go to the slaughterhouse, you would see the look of confusion and terror in their eyes. They do not know what is happening, but they do sense that it is nothing good.

Just because animals do not have a voice does not mean that they do not know the difference between right and wrong. If they could talk, they would tell us that they are afraid of going to a place where they know they will never return from, or that they are in pain.

End the conversation by asking the person: "Do you honestly believe that morality is subjective?"

The answer should be a very hard NO, because no one would want to go through life without the boundaries that have been taught to us from birth.

CAN WE NOT JUST CONSUME LESS MEAT AND DAIRY?

When being confronted with something that could be life-altering, such as your doctor telling you that you have diabetes and you need to follow a specific diet, it is human nature to find loopholes to have that piece of candy, block of chocolate or cookie. The thought of cutting your favourite snacks or food out of your diet is intimidating because you are not sure you would be able to give up the 'good' stuff.

Being faced with the option of following the vegan lifestyle is no different. Many are close to frozen in fear at the thought of never eating roast chicken, pork chops, omelettes or drinking double-thick milkshakes again. When telling people that you are considering becoming a vegan, they will tell you that you need calcium that you can only get from consuming dairy, and protein, vitamins, and nutrients that only meat and fish can provide.

As we have discussed previously, consuming animal products is not as healthy as is made to believe. Our digestive systems were not designed to digest meat and our teeth are not meant to tear into the meat and chew it the way an animal in the wild would. Knowing everything you know now and having been presented with many different scenarios and examples, the choice is quite clear. Consuming animal products is not healthy and if we value our health, there should be no compromising.

I am going to sneak an example in here which should hopefully shed some light with regards to the health issue. Smoking is bad for you. The packaging tells you. The World Health Organization tells you. Your doctor tells you.

Some may argue until they are blue in the face that they are not a smoker.

"Smokers smoke up to two packs a day, and I only have one cigarette once a week when I am at the bar, enjoying a drink with my friends."

Smoking, whether one cigarette a day, a week, or a month, is still going to affect your health. All it takes is one puff to alert cancer-forming cells to activate. If you were to change the example and insert consuming animal products, the outcome is the same.

Throughout this book, I have presented you with a lot of information regarding animal agriculture and the effects it has on the environment, the oceans, and the animals. Even though you now know everything that I have thoroughly researched, we have to agree that it is up to each of us to make an ethical decision about how we want to proceed in the next step of our lives.

Yes, we could eat meat or fish only twice a week or we could use a splash of milk in our tea or coffee once a day, rather than five times a day. Instead of having eggs for breakfast every morning, we could have them once a week. No matter what we do, or what loophole we think we might find, we would still be contributing to the death and destruction of the rainforests, the oceans, the millions of innocent animals and the environment. We would still be enabling animal agriculture even if we were consuming less.

In conclusion, while eating less meat and dairy is a positive thing, it is not a solution. If someone states they are eating less meat and dairy, I would ask them what their motivation was. Usually, the answer will be because of the animal's welfare or because of environmental issues. It is important to encourage the person and praise them because they are trying to do better, which is amazing.

However, I would still say something like: "It is great that you are reducing the amount of meat and dairy you are eating for ethical reasons, but have you thought about the fact that you are still paying for animals to be exploited and slaughtered?"

STRANDED ON A DESERTED ISLAND

"What happens if you are stranded on a deserted island, lost in the middle of the ocean, or the desert? What will you eat?" This is something which I hear quite often.

People will stop at nothing to find ways to show you that following a vegan lifestyle is not feasible. In a life or death situation, a vegan would value their own lives over that of animals. So often we hear people say: "I would never do this or that, even if it was the last option available." The truth is, people should never say that because there comes a time, for the sake of survival, that they would have to do something they never thought they would have to do.

For the sake of the argument, if I ended up being stranded on an island, I would try and find edible plants first. If there were animals on the island, there are likely to be edible plants. In all honesty, if I crawled out of the sea onto the secluded beach of an island, food is the last thing I would be thinking about. I would look for a source of fresh water. Again, if the island has trees and plants, there should be freshwater. I would then look for shelter, gather up twigs and palm tree leaves, and build a temporary structure to protect me from the elements of nature.

Andes Plane Crash

On October 12, 1972, a chartered flight carrying 45 passengers, including the crew, struck a mountain and crashed. The wreckage of the plane was found close to the Chilean border in the remote Andes Mountain range. Of the 45 passengers, 19 were members of the Old Christians Club rugby team. On impact, three crew members and eight passengers died. Due to the extreme cold and injuries sustained, several more died soon afterward. A search began, looking for survivors but after eight days, the search was called off. Over the course of 72 days, 13 passengers passed away.

When the plane went down, they had a minuscule amount of rations which included chocolate bars, jars of jam, a tin of mussels, candies, dried plums, a few dates, a tin of almonds, and several bottles of wine. They tried to make their rations last longer by portioning out small amounts. One of the survivors remembers eating a chocolate-covered peanut for three days to make it last.

No matter what they did, or how they rationed out their supplies, the food would not last forever. As they were stuck in the mountains, there was no vegetation or animals. Desperate for food, they tried to eat the cotton inside the seats, as well as the leather. Cotton and leather are treated with chemicals, and they became sicker and weaker.

They knew that they needed to eat or they would die of starvation. They were faced with the option of eating the flesh of those who had died. They agonized, some prayed for guidance, and then the remaining survivors collectively decided to eat the flesh of their dead friends, classmates, or relatives. One of the survivors set the example by consuming the frozen flesh. Some followed his example, but others could not. The following day, more tried and some refused, and some could not keep it down. To make it 'easier' to consume the flesh, they dried it in the sun.

As the flesh supply dwindled, they were forced to eat the heart, lungs, and brains.

After 72 days on December 23, 1972, all 16 remaining survivors were rescued. This tragic, yet heroic will to survive has been made into a television movie, as well as biographies by some of the survivors.

Lost in the Sahara Desert

In another story about survival, albeit not under the same circumstances of the Andes plane crash, Mauro Prosperi got lost in the Sahara Desert in 1994. Prosperi, an Italian policeman, was an athlete and long-distance runner. He participated in the Marathon of the Sands in Morocco.

While participating in the six-day race, Prosperi encountered a sandstorm that made him get lost. He ended up in an abandoned Muslim shrine in Algeria. For the sake of survival, he drank his urine, sucked the water out of wet wipes, licked dew off the rocks and ate bats. When he had given up hope of being found, he slit his wrists, but thanks to the heat, his blood clotted.

He went back into the desert and walked for nine days, eating insects and reptiles. He eventually found a villager who sent for help and he was transferred to a hospital. Upon arrival, the doctors discovered that his liver had almost failed. During this ordeal, Prosperi lost 35 pounds and it took months before he was able to eat proper food again.

The reality is, what we would do to survive cannot be compared to everyday life. We are not stuck on a deserted island, we are not sitting on a mountain top, nor are we lost in a desert. We live in a world with an abundance of vegan food choices. The bottom line is, we do not need to kill animals to survive.

ISN'T BEING A VEGETARIAN SUFFICIENT TO THE CAUSE?

People may argue that they are supporting the cause, as they have cut out eating meat for ethical reasons. Most vegetarians still consume eggs and milk. While it is a good start to the vegan lifestyle, many vegetarians do not understand the pain and torture the animals go through for those eggs or the milk. While the intention to cut out eating animal flesh is a good start, we need to educate them a little more and help them see things a little clearer. This is an excellent opportunity to help people cross the threshold from vegetarianism into veganism.

We have discussed the dairy industry in previous sections of the book, so I will not go into detail again, but everyone needs to understand the seriousness of the exploitation that takes place in the dairy industry. Just asking people simple questions such as: "Why do you think cows give milk?" and "What happens to male calves in the dairy industry, as they cannot produce milk?" should get them thinking.

You could also ask them if they ever wondered where the eggs for their weekend breakfast come from. The conditions under which eggs are obtained are horrendous.

When the eggs have hatched, the female chicks have their beaks removed. They are then transported to laying farms where they will spend the rest of their lives. Under normal circumstances, hens would lay approximately 80 to 150 eggs a year. In the factory farming setting, they are forced to lay approximately 300 eggs a year (Clauer, 2012). In the United Kingdom alone, over 10 billion eggs are laid a year.

For every egg that is laid, the hen is put through all kinds of pain. The eggshells are created by calcium from the hen's bones. The calcium deficiency causes the hens to suffer brittle bones which are easily broken and also osteoporosis. Living in cages without room to move does not help matters, and due to the lack of exercise, they develop foot problems. When their egg-laying days are over with, or if they become diseased, they are carted off to the slaughterhouses.

We have already discussed free-range farming, in which we saw that conditions deemed humane were not all they were made out to be. Instead of chickens having their beaks removed, they are trimmed. According to the guidelines for free-range farming, all farm animals should be given access to being outdoors. Most of the hens have never seen the outdoors and the space they live in is believed to be likened to the size of an iPad. They are packed in cages and they stand on top of each other. Chicken farmers, according to the law in the United Kingdom, may have 16,000 chickens per barn, this equates to approximately 9 hens per square meter. Free-range chickens are not exempt from illnesses, and because the flooring in their cages is not sufficient, they suffer from burns due to the acidity of their feces.

Follow up by asking them if they know what happens to the male chicks in the egg industry since as they know, males cannot lay eggs?

Unfortunately, the male chicks are not nearly as privileged as the females. I say this tongue in cheek because none of these factory farming animals live a privileged life. They are doomed from the moment of conception. Male chicks are useless to the egg industry. From the moment they hatch, they are put on a conveyor belt which either sends them to the gas chamber or to industrial grinders where they are minced. Keep in mind, these are brand new babies that have not yet experienced life!

Veganism is not just about a diet. Animal cruelty takes place in all types of industries such as entertainment, cosmetics, or fashion. Congratulate the person you are talking to for their choice in eliminating meat from their diets. It is a huge notch on the belts of many vegans, but we need to take it one step further. Remind them that even though they are not eating meat, they are still contributing to the senseless abuse and slaughtering of animals to keep up the supply and demand for dairy and eggs.

VEGANS ARE NOT NICE PEOPLE, THEY ARE ANNOYING

People will argue that vegans are annoying and constantly trying to make people feel guilty for consuming animal products. I have heard excuses stating that Adolf Hitler was a vegetarian and look at the atrocities he committed against the Jews. Now, as far as I know, the vegetarian claim seems to have been debunked. It is thought that Goebbels made the statement so that people would think that Adolf Hitler was more like Mahatma Gandhi, a humanitarian and a vegetarian.

The fact of the matter is that someone's diet choices are neither here nor there. For meat-eaters to label vegetarians or vegans as bad people because of one person is ludicrous. Benito Mussolini and Joseph Stalin ate meat, and they committed unforgivable crimes. If we look at Mussolini and Stalin and judge them based on their dietary habits, then all meat-eaters would be terrible people. For the sake of creating comparisons, I feel that the slaughtering of trillions of animals for immoral and unnecessary reasons is much more in line with the behaviour of the Nazis than advocating a life where animals are treated with respect and compassion.

Overall, the argument that vegans are not nice, annoying, or opinionated based on one person's experience is ridiculous. We come across people from all walks of life who are mean, deceitful and unkind. As an example, when I was traveling around Australia, I met a woman who stated that she hated British backpackers. Does this mean I can assume that all Australian women hate British backpackers?

You could ask the person you are talking to: "Do you think it is reasonable to judge an entire demographic of people based on one experience or one single person?"

FARMERS WILL LOSE THEIR JOBS

We are on a quest to promote the vegan lifestyle. It is not our intention to take away livelihoods from the farmers. Yes, this is a sensitive topic. Most farmers and farmworkers have inherited their properties from parents, grandparents and great-grandparents. Farming is in their blood, and most farmers do not have any other skills to fall back on should their farms not succeed.

The issue is not with the farmers per se, it is with the industry that dictates what they should be doing. Farming, as we have seen multiple times throughout this book, is about the exploitation and enslavement of animals against their will. That is what we are fighting for. It is a touchy subject to speak about their livelihoods, but we want to halt the exploitation of animals sooner rather than later.

Give the person who is using this excuse an example they can visualize and imagine. Think about the period in American history when the trading of slaves was permitted. No one ever said that slavery could not be ended because the livelihood of the slave traders would be at risk. What would the slave traders be doing if they no longer traded slaves? Stand back and watch your opponent thinking about that.

If the person is still not seeing your point of view, approach the topic from another direction. I would say: "I wholeheartedly agree that the issue of the farmers' livelihood needs to be addressed. My question to you is, do you believe that animal's lives and the state of the planet are worth more than money?"

Personally, I believe that the lives of the animals and the planet are much more important than money. Many people will agree. That is why it is vital to ask them questions in a manner in which they can see a clearer picture.

Farming is often associated with animals, but there are other possibilities. Instead of using the land for rearing animals, farmers can heal their land by turning it into what it was meant for, and that is growing crops for human consumption.

If we look at one of the hundreds of diets that are floating around on the internet, you will notice that the vegetable food lists call for a larger variety of vegetables. There is money in organic vegetable farming. Transitioning to plant-based farming will take time and there might be financial implications, but there are various organizations that will offer support and financial aid during the process. The Vegan Society is one such organization that will be more than willing to lend a hand.

Nadra Nittle wrote an article for an online website called Civil Eats, where she interviewed farmers who had decided to leave the meat, egg, and dairy industry. With the help of animal welfare organizations, they were able to offer support and a lifeline when needed.

Poultry Turned Hemp Farmer

Farmer Mike Weaver, a 15-year veteran in the contract farming industry stopped farming chickens in January of 2019. Instead of shutting down his farm, he surprised his neighbours by turning to hemp farming. His plans were simple. As a CBD oil user, he decided to turn his now unused chicken houses into an industrial hemp farm. He plans to purchase the necessary equipment needed to extract the oil from the hemp. As his business grows, he will hire workers, and once successfully off the ground, he will be making more money than he was farming poultry.

Mercy for Animals

Mercy for Animals is a group that has taken it upon itself to help farmers in the animal agriculture industry. They aim to grow crops such as hydroponic lettuce, mushrooms, and hemp. The president of Mercy for Animals, Leah Garcés has put together a group of people that include investors, entrepreneurs, policymakers, and engineers. The group aims to help farmers financially. The plan is that during the first phase of the project, they want to help 10 farms break away from factory farming. Garcés realizes that it is an unrealistic expectation to turn all factory farms into plant-based farming, but by starting with this is already a step in the right direction. There are no guarantees that these 10 farmers will follow through with the transition, but if everyone worked together, they could create jobs and be constructive together.

The current economic climate is not favourable for the dairy industry. One of the oldest dairy companies, Borden Dairy Co. filed for bankruptcy on January 6, 2020. It was reported that the consumption of dairy in the United States had declined between 2015 and 2019. While the dairy industry has taken a knock, more people have turned to plant-based milk such as oat milk.

Some dairy farmers have transitioned to plant-based farming. The oldest dairy farm in California, Giacomazzi shut down production on his 125-year-old dairy farm and has started growing almonds. In 2017, a New York dairy farm, Elmhurst Dairy shut down production and started to produce vegan-friendly nut-based milk (Nittle, 2020).

At the beginning of the conversation, the person you were talking to was concerned about how the farmers would survive if they gave up on the animal farming industry. After seeing the positive changes that are taking place, it is evident that their concern is unfounded. Farmers will always be farmers, and the only difference is that instead of enslaving, profiting, killing, and mutilating animals for the sake of money, they will be able to turn their immoral business model into a moral and ethical business model.

If we are going to be honest with each other, most people don't really care that much about other people's jobs. Every single day jobs are being cut due to advanced technology, but we continue to use them.

You could ask them what they think about the large supermarkets such as Target that offer the self-checkout option to avoid the queues. "If you are so concerned about the jobs and livelihood of people, what will happen to the cashiers' jobs when they are made redundant because people can help themselves?" As the world is changing, people have to change their way of living too.

ANIMALS ARE BRED FOR A PURPOSE

The question you should ask the person using this excuse is: "Who are you to decide why an animal lives or dies?"

This is a question that comes up quite frequently in conversations where veganism is discussed and it is quite similar to the "animals should be thankful that we are giving them life" excuse. It boils down to the fact that we have taken matters into our own hands by deciding what happens to animals. We are breeding animals for their meat and by-products, for entertainment, sport, and clothing. We also breed animals for companion pets. No one asked these animals what they wanted in life because human beings have shown how little they value the lives of these animals.

Dogfighting

Dogfighting is considered a spectator 'sport' for the purpose of entertainment and financial gain. Although dogfighting has been banned in all 50 states and is a felony offense, this sport continues.

Dogs are specifically bred and trained to fight against each other. The way these dogs are trained is heart-breaking, to say the least. They are abused and ill-treated from the time they are born. Even though they are being conditioned to be aggressive, it is also in the dog's nature to protect himself.

A typical fight can last between one and two hours when one of the dogs admits defeat by being unable to fight anymore. The injuries these dogs suffer include puncture wounds, broken bones, and bruising. Most of the dogs succumb to their injuries because of shock, blood loss, infection, exhaustion, or dehydration hours or days after the event.

The spectators play a massive role in the profitability of these dog fights, which keeps the sport alive. As dogfighting is illegal, events cannot be advertised. Spectators have their ways and means of finding underground dogfighting events. By paying an entrance fee and placing bets, they are willing participants in this act of cruelty.

Dog Racing

Greyhounds were bred for the purpose of dog racing, which is a sport attended by millions of spectators across the United States. Although the sport has been banned in 40 states, there are a handful of states that still have active Greyhound racetracks. On January 1, 2021, the fate of dog racing in the state of Florida was deemed illegal.

Thousands of Greyhounds are bred each year. The main purpose for the overbreeding of these dogs was to try and create the fastest dogs. During their racing career, they are kept in confinement. Their 'homes' are cages that are hardly big enough to allow them to stand up in. They are kept in these cages for up to 23 hours a day and the only comfort they have are pieces of paper or carpet for their bedding.

The injuries suffered during their racing career range from broken legs and backs to head trauma and electrocution. Some of the injuries are irreparable and they are euthanized.

Greyhound racing is a profitable venture for breeders and trainers thanks to the support of spectators. The question was asked why the trainers would treat the dogs inhumanely, and the response was that they are forever looking at ways to reduce costs to make a profit. The owners were not interested in the welfare of their dogs, unless they made them a bundle of money at the races. If and when the dogs did not perform to the expectation of the owners or the trainers, it was decided to get rid of the dogs and breed more.

Thanks to the banning and closures of the Greyhound racetracks in 40 states of the United States, animal welfare organizations have started the process of finding loving homes for these beautiful animals where they can live out the rest of their lives in comfort.

After informing the person you are talking to of the different "bred for purpose" animal scenarios, you have given them some food for thought. They will need to digest what they have learned. Many do not know what takes place behind the scenes of these types of sports. If we go to the circus, we only see the wonderful acts that are shown to the audience. We do not know what happens during training. We do not see the drugging, shackles, or whipping.

Some questions you could follow up with are: "Do you believe that you can justify dog racing as moral because we bred the Greyhounds for this purpose?" and "Do you believe that this is something that we should continue being a part of?"

A VEGAN DIET IS RESTRICTIVE, EXTREME, AND EXPENSIVE

A vegan diet is no more restrictive than following the paleo, ketogenic, or intermittent fasting diets, or any of the other hundreds of diets out there. When I first became a vegan, I was unsure about my food options. Yes, I could drink water and live on salads and bread, but that routine would go stale very quickly.

I did a little bit of research and discovered what I could eat. The options were endless and consisted of food I had never considered trying. The vegan diet is more varied than the non-vegan diet, and there are many options we can incorporate into our diets. Before my vegan days, I had never eaten lentils or beans. I had never even heard of a 'jackfruit'. Adopting the vegan lifestyle opened my eyes to a whole world of unfamiliar foods I would never have thought of trying.

When asked if I miss eating pizza, burgers, mac and cheese, pies, yogurt, and ice cream, I tell them about the vegan options that are available to me. If my friends invite me out for a night on the town, they know to choose a restaurant that offers a varied menu to cover all dietary restrictions. After all, someone in the group might be lactose or gluten intolerant, have allergies, or have celiac disease. The point I am trying to make here is that a plant-based diet is not at all restrictive.

Extreme

I love it when people refer to vegans as extreme. I like pointing out that my life is more relaxed than it was in my meat-eating days. I am no longer responsible for the senseless murder of animals. I am now able to advocate for the animals by sharing my stories, research, and experience with everyone. No, I am not extreme.

Extreme is when a cow births and loses her baby hours later. The babies do not have time to bond with their mothers, and the mothers do not have time to mourn the loss of their babies. Extreme is when an egg is hatched and a male chick is dropped into a grinder or into a container where he is killed. Extreme is when piglets are detailed the day they are born, without anesthesia or pain medication. Extreme is killing over 56 billion land animals every year.

Expensive

This is an excuse that everybody loves to use. It is a favourite when debating why you cannot follow a specific diet. IT IS TOO EXPENSIVE. Oh, do I have an eye-opener for you. No diet, regardless of the dietary lifestyle you chose, has to be expensive. No one is telling you to go out and buy all the vegan meat alternatives and ready meals, and so forth.

The cheapest food will be legumes and grains such as lentils, beans, chickpeas and rice, and in-season vegetables. In truth, you can save a lot of money by becoming a vegan because you have eliminated the most expensive items from your diet. Those expensive items just happen to be meat, eggs, and dairy.

Supermarket chains such as Target, Tesco, Walmart, Trader Joe, and Lidl offer a selection of store-brand plant-based alternatives to meat, eggs, and dairy. The best news of all is, they are affordable.

Everyone is quick to point out the cost of this, that, and the other. People do not understand that plant-based products are not as mass-produced as hamburgers, hotdogs, jugs of milk, and cartons of eggs are. The more people buy plant-based products, the more the supply and demand will increase. When the supply and demand increase, the prices of the products will decrease.

OMNIVORES HAVE CANINE TEETH

People will gleefully tell you that they have canine teeth to tear the meat you bite into, and molars to chew the meat before swallowing. I suggest, before we point out some of the flaws in their statement, we take a closer look at the differences in the various diets of the animal kingdom. As we know, there are three main types of diets where animals are concerned. Each of these diets is unique to the animals.

Carnivores

Lions, hyenas, cheetahs, and leopards belong to the carnivore species in the animal kingdom. They eat the flesh, bones, and internal organs of their prey. Carnivores have razor-sharp teeth that are used for ripping or tearing into the flesh of other animals. These teeth are known as incisors which are commonly referred to as the canines. Carnivores must catch and kill their prey before they can be eaten. They have large temporalis muscles which control the jaw. The muscles pull the lower jaw towards the skull in upward and backward motions.

Herbivores

Elephants, rhinos, hippos, and cows belong to the herbivore species in the animal kingdom. These animals live on plants. Some will eat species-specific plants. For example, koala bears will only eat eucalyptus plants, and the billy goat will eat whatever plant he comes across. Where the carnivores have razor-sharp canine teeth, most herbivores have either none or limited canines. Herbivorous animals have molars that are used to grind their food such as leaves, branches, or grass. Most herbivores have ridged molars, and their jaws move from side to side when they are chewing their food. In the cases where herbivores do have incisors, they are used to break or tear down large or difficult vegetation and it is important to note that the canines are not used to chew the food.

Omnivores

Raccoons, bears, and foxes make up the omnivore species in the animal kingdom. Omnivores consume a diet based on a mixture of plants and animals, and they can adapt their diets around the types of food which are freely available. Human beings are likened to omnivores because of the ability we possess to eat a varied diet of animal flesh and plants. We use our incisors and canines to tear the meat and our molars for chewing.

If someone were to bring up that because humans have canine teeth, we have a right to eat meat, subtly remind them that the hippopotamus has the largest canines. Hippos are herbivores. Food for thought.

Follow by asking them: "Do you believe, just because you have canine teeth, that gives you the right to unnecessarily kill animals?"

What it all boils down to is, human beings cannot be compared to an animal or any of the animal categories that have been mentioned here. We do not use our teeth to kill our prey. We do not use our teeth to tear into the flesh of an animal, nor do we use our teeth to pull a clump of grass out of the ground.

There is absolutely no comparison. What we are doing, by supporting the exploitation of animals for personal preferences, is unethical and morally wrong.

If they still insist that as omnivores, we should eat meat, then politely inform them that we do not need to eat animal products. Living off a plant-based diet will provide us with sufficient nutrients to live a long, prosperous and healthy life.

End the conversation by asking: "Just because we have the physical ability to do something, does that mean we should do it?"

FRIENDS AND FAMILY WILL NOT APPROVE OF MY VEGAN LIFESTYLE

As the caring human beings that we are, we are always looking for approval from others. We are constantly in a battle with ourselves to please everyone, regardless of what that means for us or our happiness. By now, the person you are talking to is hopefully teetering on the edge of joining the ranks of the vegan community.

It is for this reason that I wrote this book. I wanted to be able to create a visionary portal where together, we could open the eyes of our family and friends. This book was created to put you in a position where you have answers to every comment, whether genuine or snide, to win them over to transition to the vegan way of life. I am proud to say that we have given the people we have spoken to more information and explanations than they expected.

Inform the person using this excuse, that they need to help their family understand where they are coming from. If they are still living at home with their parents, it could be difficult watching them consume meat and dairy.

Their families might see their quest for veganism as a passing phase, because they believe that they cannot give up on the fried chicken from their favourite fast-food restaurant or the frozen yogurt from their favourite creamery. If they want their family to understand, they will need to explain it to them. This is a practice that will take a lot of convincing and they will encounter resistance, but they should not give up. Before long, their family will see that they are serious about the changes they are making to their lifestyle, as well as to their health.

A good way of convincing family members is by offering to cook for them. They might be sceptical about vegan food, but this is an opportunity to show everyone that plant-based food is delicious.

Another option would be to Invite family members to watch documentaries surrounding the exploitation and unethical practices of factory farming. It will educate them about the suffering that takes place, the effects animal agriculture has on the environment, and the effects that eating animal products have on their health.

If this book has been a help to you, then you could always recommend them purchasing this book to help them get their point across. They could leave it lying around, where family and friends can read through all the information that I have provided you with.

If someone is feeling pressured by their family or friends about their vegan lifestyle, there is always the option of walking away. I am not going to tell anyone to end their friendship with people who do not agree with them, but some distance might make them understand how serious you are.

It is really important that you make the person using this excuse aware of the large vegan community on social media platforms, such as Facebook, YouTube and Instagram, where they can actively engage with like-minded vegans.

There is also the option of starting their own support group. All it takes is one person to open the door for others to come flocking through. Before they know it, they will have an army of new friends that share the same passion and have the same moral values.

One last attempt to get their non-vegan friends to change their minds is to invite them over for a dinner party. This is an opportunity to showcase that any of the party foods that are normally served at parties have an alternative that is better than using the meat variety. Once their friends bite into a falafel dipped in tahini sauce, they will be convinced that they are eating minia-ture meatballs in spicy mayonnaise.

Family and friends are important in our lives. It is important to us that they understand what drives our passion. We have to be realistic with our expectations and know that not everyone will change their lifestyles because we want them to. As we have mentioned, we can plant seeds. We can give them all the infor-mation we have. Even if only one in five of our friends or family members choose the vegan way of life, that is one more than there was before you started reading this book.

At the end of the day, it is better to have thousands of imperfect vegans rather than ten resilient vegans.

ONE PERSON CANNOT MAKE A DIFFERENCE

This statement or excuse hits rather close to home. If you do not try to make a change, how will you know it will not make a difference? As we have seen multiple times throughout this book, just giving someone something to think about is already a step in the right direction. As much as we would like for there to be immediate progress, we have to allow people to go through the process of elimination.

Remember, sometimes one small action can make a huge differ-ence. One drop of water in a body of water can create a ripple. One person's smile or kind words can change your whole day.

Remember that one small mosquito that buzzed all night keeping you awake? We all know that the buzzing mosquito can drive us crazy, but think about the size of the mosquito in comparison to the disturbance it is creating.

I am going to tell you about a teenager that decided to do something proactive. What she did inspired thousands of people. Greta Thunberg, a 15-year-old Swedish girl, convinced her parents to step up to the plate and make a positive change for the environment. School days saw Greta standing outside the Swedish Parliament. She was protesting by not going to school for the sake of the climate. Students from different communities were inspired by Greta to act for what they believed in.

What started off as a simple protest against climate change, turned into a huge movement. In 2018 Greta Thunberg spoke at the United Nations Climate Change Conference in Poland. In 2019, she was invited to participate at the United Nations Climate Action Summit in North America. Staying true to her quest of reducing the carbon footprint, instead of flying, she set sail to North America. In case you were wondering, Greta is a vegan, as well as her father. It is believed that her mother is almost a full vegan.

Adopting a vegan lifestyle is a huge step to help combat climate change. Each and every single day that a person decides not to consume animals and their by-products, they are making a huge difference. If you look at the following information, you will notice that one person CAN make a difference. Each day they:

- Save one animal life
- Save 4164 litres of water
- Save 18 kg of grain
- Save 3 m² of forest
- Reduce the amount of carbon dioxide by 9 kg per day

Can one vegan make a difference? I can say with confidence that you will have the person making this excuse floored. Yes, one vegan can make a difference, together we will make a difference. One step at a time. One person at a time.

"Change will not come if we wait for some other person or some other time. We are the ones we've been waiting for. We are the change that we seek."

— BARACK OBAMA

IT IS IMPOSSIBLE TO BE 100% VEGAN

This is one argument that will have your audience convinced that they have beaten you at your own game. Until now, you have enlightened everyone you spoke to with information, facts, and scenarios. I saved this one for last because I believe that this is one of the most important excuses that non-vegans will have.

As vegans, we are not trying to be saints and telling others how to live their lives. We made a commitment to something we are passionate about. Whether we watched documentaries about animal agriculture, did research, or saw graphic images, it is a choice we made. We consciously stopped consuming and using animal products. We support organizations that are campaigning to put an end to the sport of hunting wildlife for trophies, including circuses, zoos, and rodeos for the purpose of entertainment.

Yes, it is true that we cannot lead a 100% vegan life. Even though this statement is true, it does not mean that we should consume or use animal products. By following the vegan lifestyle, we are trying to prevent the exploitation of animals for the benefit of the animals, our health, and the environment. We want to give future generations a chance to enjoy the world we live in, and for which we are fighting by eliminating animal agriculture, putting a stop to the deforestation of the rainforests, and saving our oceans–in short, we want to save our planet.

Agriculture plays an important role in our daily lives. No matter which dietary lifestyle we follow, we need food to survive. In order to produce that food, animals die in the process of farming. Mice, moles, birds, and thousands of insects perish during crop production so that we can produce enough food to feed 7 billion people.

The big difference for me is, when we buy animal products, we have paid someone to intentionally harm and slaughter animals. When I purchase plant-based products, I have not. There is a big difference between intentionally harming an animal and accidentally harming an animal.

For example, if on my way to work I accidentally hit a pigeon with my car, I would feel terrible about it, but it was an accident. We cannot compare it with seeing a flock of pigeons on the road and deciding to speed up and run them over intentionally.

When we go to a supermarket and pick up a tray of eggs, add a carton of milk to our shopping baskets, and buy a piece of brisket for dinner, we are intentionally supporting animal agriculture. When we are purchasing fruit and vegetables, including plant-based foods, we are not contributing to the exploitation of animals.

The argument surrounding the fact that we cannot be 100% vegan is true, but we are minimizing the impact of animal agriculture as much as we can. Vegans are not perfect, but at least we are trying to do something positive. Non-vegans are quick to judge us and their assessment is that what we are attempting to do is not obtainable, idealistic, and not realistic.

All we can do is continue advocating for the animals and remind non-vegans that more plants are used to feed the animals than what is used to make plant-based food. Remind the person using this excuse, that if they are concerned about the animals that are culled, injured, or killed during the production and harvesting of crops, they should be vegans.

CONCLUSION

We have reached the part of the book where I must let you go. I feel confident that I have given you all the tools you need to be the best advocate for the vegan lifestyle you can be. This book is packed full of information that will be useful on your quest.

Our journey together started with a look at the history of veganism and the influential members who gave the vegan lifestyle a name. We learned about what following a vegan lifestyle means for our health and wellbeing, the animals, and the environment. We had a crash course in how to deal with difficult questions from those who are uninformed.

We have a whole section of the book dedicated to dispelling myths and misconceptions regarding the vegan lifestyle. We have 30 of the most commonly used excuses about why following the vegan lifestyle is not a good idea. Each of those excuses has been explored and presented with examples about why the vegan lifestyle is the way of the future. I am pretty confident that we have enough information to set our opponents on the right track. We have done all we could to inform them of all their options, even giving them examples of the damage that their meat-eating habits are doing to our world.

At the end of the day, we have planted and watered the seeds for thought. It is up to everyone to decide the way forward. The changes might not happen overnight. The changes might not happen in a week. We must practice patience and play the waiting game. I know that everyone will be reminded of all we have presented them with when they next drink milk in their tea, eat a hamburger, or sit down with their bacon and egg breakfast.

Before I end this book with a final story about my friends Belinda and Stacey, I want to thank you for purchasing my book. I hope you have enjoyed reading it as much as I have enjoyed writing it.

If you found it helpful, please remember to leave a review, as your feedback is most important to me and will help other readers decide whether to purchase this book.

And now my final story:

Running up the steps from the underground station, out of breath and panting for air, I join Belinda and Stacey at the coffee shop.

"Sorry, I'm late!" I gasp.

"No worries," Belinda says, handing me a cup of coffee. "we got you a coconut milk latte. We hope that is okay with you."

"Oh!" I exclaim, slightly confused. "I've never had coconut milk in my coffee before, but I will give it a try," I say with a warm smile.

"Coconut milk is the best for lattes, in my opinion. I use oat milk for a decent cup of tea," Stacey says while sipping her coffee.

"Really? I think I just prefer soy or almond milk myself," Belinda says thoughtfully.

I stare at my two friends, slightly gob-smacked, "What are you two on about?" I ask looking from one to the other. "Since when do you guys drink oat and almond milk?" I ask, slightly dazed.

"Well, your story about the "cat milk" really got me thinking and somehow, I just cannot bring myself to drink cow's milk anymore," Stacy responds, pulling a face.

"Wait a minute, have I managed to convert you both to go vegan?" I ask with excitement.

"No! Don't push it, Lee. I have just given up dairy for now," Stacey says while stirring her latte.

"For now!" I say, turning away and feeling a grin of victory spread across my face, as I quietly think to myself. "The seed has been planted."

A FREE GIFT FOR MY READERS:

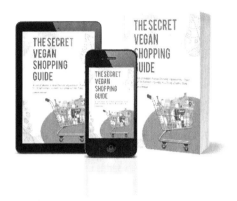

The Secret Vegan Shopping Guide

A list of hidden animal derived ingredients - from food to fashion – to help you shop cruelty fee.

Learn the truth about animal derived ingredients in your food, cosmetic products and clothing.

Could there be fish guts in your wine or animal urine in your moisturizer?

Download your free copy today and learn what ingredients you really should avoid!

Visit this link to get your copy for free:

www.the-vegan-club.com

REFERENCES

19 vegan quotes [quotations that make you think] -. (2015, March 19). VegInspired. https://www.veginspired.com/19-vegan-quotes-quotations-that-make-you-think

A quote from Lady Oracle. (n.d.). Www.goodreads.com. https://www.goodreads.com/quotes/815563-if-you-can-t-say-anything-nice-don-t-say-anything-at

Admin. (2016, February 23). Lives lost to leather: Toxic chemicals harming child workers in Bangladesh. Trusted Clothes. https://www.trustedclothes.com/blog/2016/02/23/24811/

American Cancer Society. (n.d.). Known and probable human carcinogens. Cancer.org; American Cancer Society. https://www.cancer.org/cancer/cancer-causes/general-info/known-and-probable-human-carcinogens.html

Amnesty International. (2019, November 26). Amnesty International. Amnesty.org. https://www.amnesty.org/en/latest/news/2019/11/brazil-halt-illegal-cattle-farms-fuelling-amazon-rainforest-destruction/

Animals used for food | PETA. (n.d.). PETA. https://www.peta.org/issues/animals-used-for-food/

BBC. (2020, January 6). Confessions of a slaughterhouse worker. BBC News. https://www.bbc.com/news/stories-50986683

BDA. (2017, August 7). British Dietetic Association confirms well-planned vegan diets can support healthy living in people of all ages. Www.bda.uk.com. https://www.bda.uk.com/resource/british-dietetic-association-confirms-well-planned-vegan-diets-can-support-healthy-living-in-people-of-all-ages.html

Belle, C. (2021, January 31). We could see fishless oceans by 2048. Medium. https://medium.com/age-of-awareness/we-could-see-fishless-oceans-by-2048-9a2ba269887b

Bethany. (2018, August 1). Why do meat eaters get so defensive? Little Green Seedling. https://littlegreenseedling.com/2018/08/01/meat-eaters-defensive

Biswas, S., & Rahman, T. (2013). The effect of working place on worker's health in a tannery in Bangladesh. Advances in Anthropology, 03(01), 46–53. https://doi.org/10.4236/aa.2013.31007

Brighten, T. (2015, August 26). Taiji dolphin slaughter turns cove into bloodbath. Tracy Brighten. https://tracybrighten.-com/animal-welfare/taiji-dolphin-slaughter-turns-cove-into-bloodbath/

Carnivores, Omnivores, and Herbivores: Their differences and roles in the food chain. (n.d.). Www.dentalone-Md.com. https://www.dentalone-md.com/locations/oxon-hill/carni-vores-omnivores-and-herbivores-their-differences-and-roles-in-the-food-chain/

Changing Works. (n.d.). Open and closed questions. Changing-minds.org. http://changingminds.org/techniques/questioning/open_-closed_questions.htm

Clauer, P. (2012, July 5). Modern egg industry. Penn State Extension. https://extension.psu.edu/modern-egg-industry

Cole, M., & Morgan, K. (2011). Vegaphobia: Derogatory discourses of veganism and the reproduction of speciesism in UK national newspapers1. The British Journal of Sociology, 62(1), 134–153. https://doi.org/10.1111/j.1468-4446.2010.01348.x

COWSPIRACY: The Sustainability Secret. (2013). COWSPIRACY. COWSPIRACY. https://www.cowspiracy.com/facts

Creation - Revision 1 - GCSE Religious Studies - BBC Bitesize. (1 B.C.E.). BBC Bitesize. https://www.bbc.co.uk/bitesize/guides/zg3vxfr/revision/1

Dahlman, L., & Lindsey, R. (2020, August 17). Climate change: Ocean heat content | NOAA Climate.gov. Climate.gov. https://www.climate.gov/news-features/understanding-climate/climate-change-ocean-heat-content

Dalai Lama Quotes :: Quoteland :: Quotations by Author. (n.d.). Www.quoteland.com. http://www.quoteland.com/author/Dalai-Lama-Quotes/454/

Daly, N. (2019, July 4). Domesticated animals, explained. Animals. https://www.nationalgeographic.com/animals/article/domesticated-animals

Definition of CARCINOGEN. (n.d.). Merriam-Webster.com. https://www.merriam-webster.com/dictionary/carcinogen

Dei, H. (2011, August). (PDF) Soybean as a feed ingredient for livestock and poultry. ResearchGate. https://www.researchgate.net/publication/221918704_Soybean_as_a_Feed_Ingredient_for_Livestock_and_Poultry

Earthling Ed. (n.d.). 30 non-vegan excuses & how to respond to them.[1]

Earthday.org. (2019, August 8). UN report: Plant-based diets provide "major opportunities" to address climate crisis. Earth Day. https://www.earthday.org/un-report-plant-based-diets-provide-major-opportunities-to-address-climate-crisis/

EasyTeaching. (2020). What are food chains | Learning Science | EasyTeaching [YouTube Video]. In YouTube. https://www.youtube.com/watch?v=8y1GiTdQDgE

Editors, H. com. (2019, June 20). Eating bats, drinking urine: 5 stunning real-life survival stories. HISTORY. https://www.history.com/news/5-stunning-real-life-survival-stories

Enjoli, A. (2020, August 7). 19 vegan athletes who swear by plant-based diets. LIVEKINDLY. https://www.livekindly.co/vegan-athletes-swear-by-plants/

Evans, K. (2019, July 29). What kind of emotions do animals feel? Greater Good. https://greatergood.berkeley.edu/article/item/what_kind_of_emotions_do_animals_feel

familydoctor.org editorial staff. (2020, July 31). Vegan diet: How to get the nutrients you need - familydoctor.org. Familydoctor.org. https://familydoctor.org/vegan-diet-how-to-get-the-nutrients-you-need/

Food Allergy Research & Education. (n.d.). Soy. Food Allergy Research & Education. https://www.foodallergy.org/living-food-allergies/food-allergy-essentials/common-allergens/soy

Forrest, C. (2020, August 9). Potential risks of a vegan diet (One is irreversible) - Clean eating kitchen. Clean Eating Kitchen. https://www.cleaneatingkitchen.com/vegan-diet-dangers-health/#Eight_Potential_Vegan_Diet_Dangers

Geoff Watts. (2019, August 7). The cows that could help fight climate change. Bbc.com; BBC Future. https://www.bbc.-com/future/article/20190806-how-vaccines-could-fix-our-problem-with-cow-emissions

Gleerup, K. B. (2018). Assessing pain in horses. In Practice, 40(10), 457–463. https://doi.org/10.1136/inp.k4781

Good, K. (2015, January 22). Explain like I'm 5: Why tofu consumption is not responsible for soy-related deforestation. One Green Planet; One Green Planet. https://www.onegreen-planet.org/environment/why-tofu-consumption-is-not-respon-sible-for-soy-related-deforestation/

Hagan, E. (2011, November 17). Was Hitler a vegetarian? The Nazi Animal Protection Movement. Psychology Today. https://www.psychologytoday.com/za/blog/animals-and-us/201111/was-hitler-vegetarian-the-nazi-animal-protection-movement

Head, T. (2018, November 9). SPCA hunt for "heartless" driver who deliberately ran over baby ducklings. The South African. https://www.thesouthafrican.com/news/spca-cape-town-driver-ducklings/

Hickman, M. (2011, October 22). Study claims meat creates half of all greenhouse gases. The Independent. https://www. independent.co.uk/climate-change/news/study-claims-meat-creates-half-of-all-greenhouse-gases-1812909.html

History.com Editors. (2018, August 27). Slavery in America. HISTORY. https://www.history.com/topics/black-history/slavery#section_2

Humane Slaughter Association. (n.d.). General - Humane Slaughter Association. Hsa.org.uk. https://www.h-sa.org.uk/faqs/general

Humane Society International. (2016, March 21). Cruel Kots Kaal Pato Festival in Yucatan, Mexico to end. Humane Society International. https://www.hsi.org/news-media/yucatan-cruel-kots-kaal-pato-festival-to-end-032116/

Hume, D. (2018, July 29). Ocean storage of CO2. The Maritime Executive. https://www.maritime-executive.com/features/ocean-storage-of-co2

Hutyra, H. (2017, April 13). 119 Socrates quotes that offer a more peaceful way of life. KeepInspiring.me. https://www.-keepinspiring.me/socrates-quotes/

IARC working group on the evaluation of carcinogenic risk to humans. (2018). Red meat and processed Meat. Nih.gov; International Agency for Research on Cancer. https://www.

ncbi.nlm.nih.gov/books/NBK507971/

Jenn Sinrich. (2019, October 3). 10 things that happen to your body if you stop eating red meat. The Healthy; The Healthy. https://www.thehealthy.com/nutrition/stop-eating-red-meat/

Kamal, B. (2017, August 21). Climate migrants might reach one billion by 2050 | Inter Press Service. Ipsnews.net. http://www.ipsnews.net/2017/08/climate-migrants-might-reach-one-billion-by-2050/

Krauss Whitbourne, S. (2014, August 16). 6 ways to win any argument. Psychology Today. https://www.psychologytoday.com/us/blog/fulfillment-any-age/201408/6-ways-win-any-argument

Lemony Snicket Quote: "Just because something is traditional is no reason to do it, of course." (n.d.). Quotefancy.com.

Lin, D. (2019, November 25). As vegans know, animal products cannot be strictly avoided. Treehugger. https://www.treehugger.com/is-there-no-such-thing-as-vegan-127588

Lingel, G. (2018). Veganism: 20 powerful reasons you should go vegan. In sentientmedia.org. https://sentientmedia.org/veganism/

Linnekin, B. J. (2017, May 2). "America's slaughterhouse mess." The Counter. https://thecounter.org/americas-slaughterhouse-mess/

Lupica, D. (2018, January 5). Oceanic dead zones quadruple since 1950 due to animal agriculture, scientists warn. Plant Based News. https://plantbasednews.org/news/oceanic-dead-zones-increased-1000-1950-animal-agriculture-new-study/

Madisha, L. (n.d.). Difference between pet and domestic animals | Difference between. http://www.differencebetween.net/science/nature/difference-between-pet-and-domestic-animals/

Maier, C. (2018, April 25). The effects of animal overpopulation. Sciencing. https://sciencing.com/effects-animal-overpopulation-8249633.html

Main Street Children's Dentistry & Orthodontics. (n.d.). Dental and skull anatomy of carnivores, herbivores, and omnivores. Www.mainstreetsmiles.com. https://www.mainstreetsmiles.com/dental-and-skull-anatomy-of-carnivores-herbivores-and-omnivores/

McEvoy, M. (2019, March 13). Organic 101: What the USDA organic label means. Usda.gov. https://www.usda.gov/media/blog/2012/03/22/organic-101-what-usda-organic-label-means

McLaughlin, S. (2021, January 28). The 30 best vegan food finds at Walmart: The ultimate guide. VegNews.com. https://vegnews.com/2021/1/best-vegan-food-walmart

McManus, K. (2018, September 27). What is a plant-based diet and why should you try it? - Harvard Health Blog. Harvard Health Blog. https://www.health.harvard.edu/blog/what-is-a-plant-based-diet-and-why-should-you-try-it-2018092614760

Nittle, N. (2020, January 13). The plant-based movement to transition farmers away from meat and dairy production. Civil eats. https://civileats.com/2020/01/13/the-plant-based-move-ment-to-transition-farmers-away-from-meat-and-dairy-production/

Oscar. (2021, February 10). What does free range really mean? - Greener choices. Greener Choices. https://www.greenerchoic-es.org/free-range/

Parsons, R. (2020, August 7). 10 Phenomenal reasons to love pigs. One Green Planet. https://www.onegreenplanet.org/ani-malsandnature/phenomenal-reasons-to-love-pigs/

PETA. (n.d.-a). All about PETA | PETA. PETA. https://www.peta.org/about-peta/learn-about-peta/

PETA. (n.d.-b). Animals used for clothing | PETA. PETA. https://www.peta.org/issues/animals-used-for-clothing/

PETA. (n.d.-c). Animals used for entertainment | PETA. PETA. https://www.peta.org/issues/animals-in-entertainment/

Petruzzello, M. (n.d.). Do plants feel pain? | Britannica. In Encyclopædia Britannica. https://www.britannica.com/story/do-plants-feel-pain

Plant Based News LTD. (2019, February 11). What is veganism? Academy.plantbasednews.org. https://academy.plantbasednews.org/blog/what-is-veganism

Poore, J., & Nemecek, T. (2018). Reducing food's environmental impacts through producers and consumers. Science, 360(6392), 987–992. https://doi.org/10.1126/science.aaq0216

Riddell, K. (2020, May 1). Three men charged with breaking lockdown and beating duck to death. ChronicleLive. https://www.chroniclelive.co.uk/news/north-east-news/county-durham-duck-killed-police-18183652

Robinson, L., Segal, J., & Smith, M. (2019, March 21). Effective communication. HelpGuide.org. https://www.helpguide.org/articles/relationships-communication/effective-communication.htm

Sebastiani, G., Herranz Barbero, A., Borrás-Novell, C., Alsina Casanova, M., Aldecoa-Bilbao, V., Andreu-Fernández, V., Pascual Tutusaus, M., Ferrero Martínez, S., Gómez Roig, M., & García-Algar, O. (2019). The effects of vegetarian and vegan diet during pregnancy on the health of mothers and offspring. Nutrients, 11(3), 557. https://doi.org/10.3390/nu11030557

Shutler, Dr. J., & Watson, Prof. A. (2020, September 28). Guest post: The oceans are absorbing more carbon than previously thought. Carbon Brief. https://www.carbonbrief.org/guest-post-the-oceans-are-absorbing-more-carbon-than-previously-thought

Sicinski, A. (n.d.). Are you living a life of endless excuses? Here's how to stop! IQ Matrix Blog. https://blog.iqmatrix.com/a-life-of-excuses

Steber, C. (2017, June 22). 11 Ways to win any argument, no matter what. Bustle. https://www.bustle.com/p/11-ways-to-win-any-argument-no-matter-what-64435

Sterk, R. (2020, May 15). Meat prices expected to rise as supply continues to decrease. Www.meatpoultry.com. https://www.meatpoultry.com/articles/23131-meat-prices-expected-to-rise-as-supply-continues-to-decrease

SURGE CAMPAIGNING C.I.C. (n.d.). SURGE | Why should I go vegan? SURGE. https://www.surgeactivism.org/whyvegan

The Associated Press. (2018, October 5). Quote wrongly attributed to Mahatma Gandhi. AP NEWS. https://apnews.com/article/2315880316

The Game Changers Movie. (n.d.). The Game Changers movie. The Game Changers Movie. https://gamechangersmovie.com/the-film/

The Happy Chicken Coop. (n.d.). A history of chickens: Then (1900) vs now (2016). Thehappychickencoop.com. https://www.thehappychickencoop.com/a-history-of-chickens/

The Humane Society of the United States. (n.d.-a). Animal cruelty and neglect FAQ. The Humane Society of the United States. https://www.humanesociety.org/resources/animal-cruelty-and-neglect-faq#criminal

The Humane Society of the United States. (n.d.). Dogfighting fact sheet. The Humane Society of the United States. https://www.humanesociety.org/resources/dogfighting-fact-sheet

The Humane Society of the United States. (n.d.-b). Greyhound racing FAQ. The Humane Society of the United States. https://www.humanesociety.org/resources/greyhound-racing-faq

The truth about soy - Busting the myths. (2016, February 27). RiseOfTheVegan.com. https://www.riseofthevegan.com/blog/the-truth-about-soy-busting-the-myths

The Vegan Society. (n.d.). History. The Vegan Society. https://www.vegansociety.com/about-us/history

Top 25 one person can make a difference quotes (of 52). (n.d.). A-Z Quotes. https://www.azquotes.com/quotes/topics/one-person-can-make-a-difference.html

Toro de la Vega. (2021, January 25). Wikipedia. https://en.wikipedia.org/wiki/Toro_de_la_Vega

US - Slaughter - Humane slaughter of livestock regulations | Animal legal & historical center. (2020, March). Www.animallaw.info. https://www.animallaw.info/administrative/us-slaughter-humane-slaughter-livestock-regulations

Vegan Calculator. (n.d.). 5 Vegan. https://www.5vegan.org/tools/vegan-save-calculator/

Von Alt, S. (2017, May 24). The vegan's guide to talking with meat eaters. ChooseVeg. https://chooseveg.com/blog/heres-how-to-have-a-conversation-about-veganism/

Wartenberg, L. (2020, May 25). Raw or undercooked pork: Risks and side effects to know. Healthline. https://www.healthline.com/nutrition/raw-pork-or-undercooked-pork

Watson, C. P. (2018, March 19). If the ocean dies, we all die! Sea Shepherd. https://seashepherd.org/2015/09/29/if-the-ocean-dies-we-all-die/

What does Genesis 9:4 mean? (n.d.). BibleRef.com. https://www.bibleref.com/Genesis/9/Genesis-9-4.html

Whittleton, J. (2018, November 22). The heartbreaking story behind intensive pig breeding | World Animal Protection. Www.worldanimalprotection.org. https://www.worldanimalprotection.org/blogs/heartbreaking-story-behind-intensive-pig-breeding

Wikipedia Contributors. (2018, November 23). Uruguayan air force flight 571. Wikipedia; Wikimedia Foundation. https://en.wikipedia.org/wiki/Uruguayan_Air_Force_Flight_571

Wikipedia Contributors. (2019a, February 5). Socrates. Wikipedia; Wikimedia Foundation. https://en.wikipedia.org/wiki/Socrates

Wikipedia Contributors. (2019b, March 18). Greta Thunberg. Wikipedia; Wikimedia Foundation. https://en.wikipedia.org/wiki/Greta_Thunberg

Wikipedia Contributors. (2019c, March 18). Socratic method. Wikipedia; Wikimedia Foundation. https://en.wikipedia.org/wiki/Socratic_method

Wikipedia Contributors. (2019d, October 3). Lychee and dog meat festival. Wikipedia; Wikimedia Foundation. https://en.wikipedia.org/wiki/Lychee_and_Dog_Meat_Festival

Wikipedia Contributors. (2019e, November 10). Slaughterhouse. Wikipedia; Wikimedia Foundation. https://en.wikipedia.org/wiki/Slaughterhouse

Wikipedia Contributors. (2019f, December 3). Cowspiracy. Wikipedia; Wikimedia Foundation. https://en.wikipedia.org/wiki/Cowspiracy

William Butler Yeats Quotes. (n.d.). BrainyQuote. https://www.brainyquote.com/quotes/william_butler_yeats_133805

World Animal Foundation. (2021, April 14). Veganism can end world hunger. Worldanimalfoundation.com. https://www.worldanimalfoundation.com/advocate/farm-animals/params/post/1280889/veganism-can-end-world-hunger

World, G. (2013, August 7). Veganism defined (written by Leslie Cross, 1951). Gentle World. https://gentleworld.org/veganism-defined-written-by-leslie-cross-1951/

Yip, C. (2018, August 2). What do newspapers say about vegans? Faunalytics. https://faunalytics.org/what-do-newspapers-say-about-vegans/

Printed in Great Britain
by Amazon